FIRST STEPS IN
COGNITIVE
BEHAVIOUR
THERAPY

T0323209

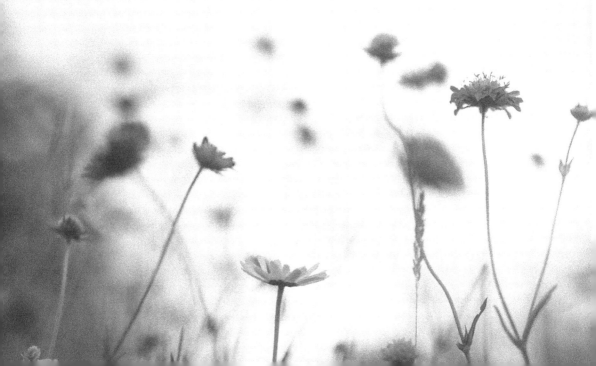

Sara Miller McCune founded SAGE Publishing in 1965 to support the dissemination of usable knowledge and educate a global community. SAGE publishes more than 1000 journals and over 800 new books each year, spanning a wide range of subject areas. Our growing selection of library products includes archives, data, case studies and video. SAGE remains majority owned by our founder and after her lifetime will become owned by a charitable trust that secures the company's continued independence.

Los Angeles | London | New Delhi | Singapore | Washington DC | Melbourne

FIRST STEPS IN

COGNITIVE BEHAVIOUR THERAPY

SARAH CORRIE
DAVID A. LANE

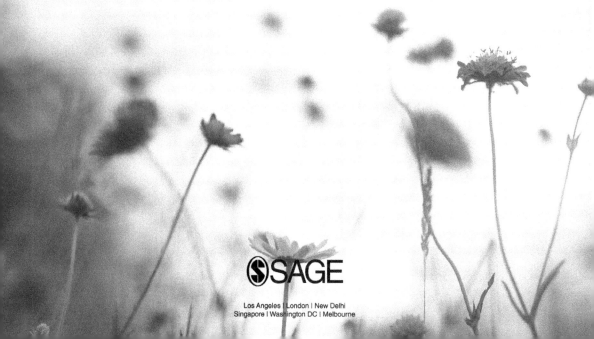

$SAGE

Los Angeles | London | New Delhi
Singapore | Washington DC | Melbourne

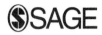

Los Angeles | London | New Delhi
Singapore | Washington DC | Melbourne

SAGE Publications Ltd
1 Oliver's Yard
55 City Road
London EC1Y 1SP

SAGE Publications Inc.
2455 Teller Road
Thousand Oaks, California 91320

SAGE Publications India Pvt Ltd
B 1/I 1 Mohan Cooperative Industrial Area
Mathura Road
New Delhi 110 044

SAGE Publications Asia-Pacific Pte Ltd
3 Church Street
#10-04 Samsung Hub
Singapore 049483

Editor: Susannah Trefgarne
Assistant editor: Ruth Lilly
Production editor: Rachel Burrows
Copyeditor: Sarah Bury
Proofreader: Brian McDowell
Indexer: Gary Kirby
Marketing manager: Dilhara Attygalle
Cover design: Naomi Robinson
Typeset by: KnowledgeWorks Global Ltd.
Printed in the UK

Library of Congress Control Number: 2020947333

British Library Cataloguing in Publication data

A catalogue record for this book is available from the
British Library

ISBN 978-1-5264-9917-2
ISBN 978-1-5264-9916-5 (pbk)

At SAGE we take sustainability seriously. Most of our products are printed in the UK using responsibly
sourced papers and boards. When we print overseas we ensure sustainable papers are used as measured
by the PREPS grading system. We undertake an annual audit to monitor our sustainability.

Contents

List of Figures, Tables and Reflective Activities

Figures

Tables

Reflective Activities

About the Authors

Sarah Corrie is a Chartered Psychologist, Consultant Clinical Psychologist and Accredited Therapist, Supervisor and Trainer with the British Association for Behavioural & Cognitive Psychotherapies (BABCP). Her work as a CBT scholar is extensive and spans innovations in practice, training and supervision. Formerly a programme director of courses delivered by The Central London CBT Training Centre at CNWL NHS Foundation Trust, Sarah was also a member of CNWL's Leadership and Training Team to support the national expansion and dissemination of behavioural couple therapy as part of the 'Improving Access to Psychological Therapies' initiative. She is also currently Chair of the BABCP's Course Accreditation Committee.

Sarah has authored over 80 articles for academic journals, professional journals and trade magazines as well as eight books. The most recent of these is a co-authored text on CBT for couples – *Treating Relationship Distress and Psychopathology in Couples: A Cognitive-Behavioural Approach* (Routledge). She also co-wrote and edited the second edition of *Assessment and Case Formulation in Cognitive Behavioural Therapy*.

A Visiting Professor at Middlesex University and a faculty member of the Professional Development Foundation, one of Sarah's main interests is supporting the learning and development needs of the workforce and establishing practices that support the well-being of mental health professionals.

As a Registered Coaching Psychologist, she is a Founder Member and former Chair of the British Psychological Society's Special Group in Coaching Psychology and has a particular interest in how coaching might contribute to some of the most challenging issues of our time, including emotional well-being and mental health.

In 2016, she was the recipient of the British Psychological Society's Achievement Award for Distinguished Contributions to Coaching Psychology and in 2017 was awarded a Fellowship of the British Association for Behavioural & Cognitive Psychotherapies for her contribution to CBT training and supervision. In 2020, Sarah was appointed Visiting Professor in Cognitive Behaviour Therapy and Counselling at the University of Suffolk.

David A. Lane is Director and co-founder of the Professional Development Foundation, which has for forty years pioneered work-based professional development. As well as contributing to research and professional development in counselling psychology and coaching, David has worked in a wide range of organisations, including major consultancies, multinationals, and public sector and government bodies. He is a Visiting Professor at both Middlesex University and Canterbury Christ Church University.

David was Chair of the British Psychological Society Register of Psychologists Specialising in Psychotherapy and convened the European Federation of Psychologists Association's group on Psychotherapy. He established the first behaviour support service to work across school systems as part of the Inner London Education Authority in 1975. This service was research based and pioneered the use of many behavioural and later cognitive behavioural approaches. He developed an individualised approach to case formulation. While running this service he also worked with Vic Meyer and Ted Chessor at Middlesex Hospital where they had established a behaviour therapy ward. For more than 20 years David taught case formulation to students at that clinic. David was a member of the BABP (later BACBP) from that time and active in the Association for Behavioural Approaches with Children.

David's contributions to counselling psychology led to the senior award of the British Psychological Society (BPS) for 'Outstanding Scientific Contribution'. In 2009 he received the award for Distinguished Contribution to Professional Psychology from the BPS. In 2016 he became an Honorary Associate of the Royal College of Veterinary Surgeons (their highest award to a non-vet) in recognition of the work establishing education in general practice. He is also a Fellow of the Academy of Social Sciences for contributions to education. In 2018 he received a Lifetime Achievement Award from the University of Surrey. The Association of Professional Executive Coaches and Supervisors made him a Fellow in 2020.

Acknowledgements

There are a number of people who have contributed to the development of this book and whose interest, encouragement and support we wish to acknowledge.

First, we would like to thank Susannah Trefgarne and the team at SAGE who have been such supportive and enthusiastic partners. We have greatly valued this latest opportunity to work with SAGE.

Second, we thank all of those scholars – researchers, practitioners, teachers and supervisors – whose work over the years has shaped our understanding of cognitive behaviour therapy and our commitment to this way of working. Their influence has profoundly impacted how we listen to clients, help them arrive at an understanding of themselves and their needs, and develop effective and ethical practices.

Third, as much, or perhaps more, gratitude is owed to all the clients whose journeys we have had the privilege of sharing. Learning from the experience of working with clients has been central for both of us in building our approaches to therapy. Each of us has worked with different clients and has trained across varied client groups. Learning from each other has been an essential process in testing our ideas and has been a great pleasure.

We also offer thanks to our colleagues at the Professional Development Foundation, Middlesex University, Christ Church Canterbury University and more recently the University of Chester, as well as our students who have accepted our invitation to learn together and influenced our thinking in many ways.

Sarah Corrie wishes to acknowledge her current and former students and colleagues for their inspiration and guidance and from whom she has learned so much. Thanks also go to her colleagues at the British Association for Behavioural & Cognitive Psychotherapy and, in particular, her colleagues on the Course Accreditation Committee for their wisdom, support and contribution to advancing the specialism of CBT training and supervision.

David A. Lane wishes to acknowledge colleagues at University College Hospital, particularly the late Ted Chesser and Vic Meyer for their inspiration, and Mary Watts and Michael Bruch, with whom he has shared his journey in CBT for many years. All his colleagues at the Islington Educational Guidance Centre and other Behaviour Support Teams throughout the UK have supported him through their active participation as he explored various approaches to developing services. Special thanks to Fiona Green, who is a constant companion on the journey, and to Julius Malkin and Peggy Gosling, who carried the banner forward.

Finally, special thanks go to Ian Lacey for proofreading the manuscript and for his encouragement, critique and unfailing belief in the project and its authors.

Praise for the Book

'Corrie and Lane's *First Steps in Cognitive Behaviour Therapy* outlines the basic concepts, techniques and widening applications of the most empirically validated form of psychotherapy. It is well written and easy to understand. The authors, both highly respected leaders in the field, have produced one the most accessible texts on the subject that I have ever had the pleasure of reading. A valuable resource with wide appeal to anyone interested in learning about CBT from the simply curious to HR practitioners, coaches and students.'

Dr Marc Kahn, Global Head of People and Organisation, Investec Plc and Visiting Professor, Middlesex University. Author of Coaching on the Axis: Working with Complexity in Business and Executive Coaching

'Sarah Corrie and David Lane present the first steps in CBT with remarkable and consistent clarity even when dealing with relatively complex topics. In my opinion, this is an excellent introduction to CBT and will be enjoyed by many students and trainees entering this field.'

Stuart Turner, MD MA FRCP FRCPsych Trauma Clinic London & Past President, International Society for Traumatic Stress Studies

'I've spent many years as a CBT practitioner and read many books on the subject and for me this one really stands out. Why? – Because from the very start the authors of *First Steps in Cognitive Behaviour Therapy* form a relationship with the reader supporting their learning and understanding from beginning to end.

Whether you are an experienced or novice therapist, a coach, a professional from a completely different context, a potential or actual client, or none of these, the book is written in a way that all can relate to and apply to their own unique life – past, present and future.

This is a shorter book than many on the subject, and I suspect that once you start reading it you won't want to put it down. What could be complex and dry material is presented in a powerful, lively, simple (but far from simplistic) way, and it cannot fail to touch its readers in ways that impact on their own lives and also others with whom they interact professionally or personally. I unreservedly recommend this book by Sarah Corrie and David Lane.'

Professor Mary Watts, Emeritus Professor of Psychology, City, University of London

'This is an excellently well-written book, which introduces the history, key scientific and philosophical underpinnings; principles and practice of cognitive-behaviour therapy (CBT). The style is thoughtful and engaging. The authors achieve a sound balance of explaining concepts in a way which does not assume prior knowledge, but does not patronise the reader. There are illustrative examples of a range of situations which demonstrate the approaches being discussed. The book makes use of the principles described, by offering reflective learning activities, and signposting to further reading at the end of each chapter. It provides an up to date, engaging overview of the field, noting the core researchers and current developments which inform CBT. I would recommend this book to anyone starting training in CBT, as well as fundamental reading for therapists training in other orientations or schools of thought, mental health and well-being therapists, and as a core reference for CBT training programmes.'

Helen Macdonald, MBE, BABCP Chief Accred Officer

'Sarah Corrie and David Lane have provided a very timely and easy to understand book about Cognitive Behavioural Psychotherapy (CBT). The book is mainly intended for people suffering from mental disorders looking for help but also interested individuals and mental health professionals who seek knowledge regarding the workings of this scientifically developed and most successful therapeutic methodology in our time. The book informs comprehensively for those who seek help, direction and suitable professional guidance.

This book should be a very useful guide for people looking for a therapeutic approach based on scientific principles but also for health professional in training and practice for psychotherapy. It is also highly recommended for any reading list with CBT training courses.'

Michael Bruch, University College London

'This book is a new departure for Sarah and David. As highly qualified academics, they usually produce books and papers for those familiar with psychological topics. In this excellent book, they seek to help those of us less familiar with CBT to understand the principles on which it is built and the ways it is used effectively in practice.

As I should have expected, they have written a book that is easy to read without dumbing down the academic rigor. Indeed, one of its real attractions is how they have made the book very accessible by using fictitious case studies drawn from their vast experience as practitioners. In addition, there are regular prompts for the reader to self-reflect on how they might apply the contents. They end with a brief look at where CBT may develop in the future. I highly recommend this book for any non-expert or lay person who is keen to gain better understanding of CBT for their own personal or professional lives. You will not regret the time taken in allowing Sarah and David to lead you gently to a greater understanding of CBT.'

Phil Moore, GP, Mental Health Commissioner

'A beautifully written book: clear and easy to understand, and comprehensively covering the key principles and techniques of cognitive behavioural therapy. Fictional case examples bring components of CBT to life and reflective exercises provide opportunities to reflect on how to relate CBT principles to one's own life. Extremely useful for trainee cognitive behavioural therapists, and anyone interested in understanding what cognitive behavioural therapy is.'

Dr Lucy Maddox, consultant clinical psychologist and author of
Blueprint: How Our Childhood Makes Us Who We Are

A Note on Confidentiality

The case material included in this book has been inspired by dilemmas encountered in professional practice. However, care has been taken to ensure anonymity and the clients and therapists in all cases are fictitious.

Introduction

Cognitive behaviour therapy – otherwise known as CBT – has become something of a modern age phenomenon. With the introduction into health care and related disciplines of evidence-based practice, CBT, with its strong empirical foundations, is seen by many as the approach of choice for a range of human concerns. Moreover, visit the personal development section of any self-respecting book shop and you are almost certain to find a range of CBT-focused resources. Its foundational principles and methods have inspired many disciplines, including behavioural medicine, coaching, education, mental health nursing, organisational consultancy, psychiatry, psychotherapy and sports psychology, to name but a few.

The growing popularity of CBT has created both opportunities and challenges. As something of a celebrity therapy (we discovered to our surprise that it is now even possible to buy 'I love CBT' T-shirts and mugs!), it is attracting increased scrutiny from both supporters and dissenters. Inevitably, such scrutiny has at times given rise to inflated claims of effectiveness as well as myths that misrepresent the approach. The scholars who have shaped the theory and practice of CBT understand all too well the challenges of devising effective responses to human problems – indeed it is these challenges that have inspired the innovations described in the chapters that follow. However, the popularity of CBT can create confusion for those who are new to the approach and who wish to find a way to differentiate fact from fiction in order to learn more about this fascinating discipline. *First Steps in Cognitive Behaviour Therapy* aims to meet the needs of an increasing number of professionals, aspiring CBT therapists and members of the public who wish to become more informed about what CBT truly entails. It provides a practical and accessible introduction to one of the most impactful fields in mental health and applied psychology, offering a flavour of its background through key references from the past as well as sources of information relating to current practices and trends.

An introductory text like this is needed in part because CBT is such a highly diverse field. Rather than any unified approach, it is best understood as a family of therapies that encompass a wide range of concepts, principles, theories, models, methods and techniques. This breadth of perspective and approach represents part of its appeal for many. Yet this poses some significant dilemmas when it comes to writing an introductory text that seeks to provide an orientation to the field. In particular, we have had to make difficult choices about which areas to prioritise and which to signpost as topics for follow-up reading. We wanted to avoid being over-inclusive in a way which creates an impression that CBT consists of little more than an eclectic use of disunified techniques. We have also sought to avoid the trap, present in many introductory texts, of oversimplifying procedure and method for ease of understanding. Rather, it was a priority for us that we found a way to capture the richness, depth and texture of the field and to document aspects of its history so that you could put in context the wealth of methods that represent CBT today.

In attempting to provide a balanced overview of CBT, our approach has been to select the foundational principles and perspectives that underpin this family of therapies and then illustrate how they have given rise to specific categories of technique. Thus, concepts and techniques derived from behavioural and cognitive sources are introduced and then illustrated in the different chapters through their application to a variety of problems of living.

To give you a solid grounding in the fundamentals of CBT, we have chosen to organise the book in three parts. Part I familiarises you with its theoretical and conceptual foundations. Part II explores some of the most commonly used methods and techniques. Part III considers the application of CBT to therapeutic practice and beyond. This final part of the book includes a consideration of how CBT therapists use the various principles and methods to make sense of their clients' needs (also termed 'formulation') and a chapter speculating on future directions for the field in light of the increasing social and economic pressures faced by us all. Finally, in the conclusion to the book, we offer you a reflective tool to help you consolidate your thinking and learning and to help you identify any next steps that you might wish to take.

Embedded within the book are two specific learning features. The first is the use of (fictitious but representative) case material which comprises vignettes, brief clinical descriptions and segments of session transcripts. For each chapter we have selected a form of illustration which we believe reflects the principle or method that we are exploring to best advantage and which we hope will give you a sense of what participating in CBT looks and feels like.

The second learning feature is the use of a self-reflective exercise at the end of each chapter to help you consider how you might apply the content to an area of your personal or your professional life. The field of CBT is committed to experiential learning (i.e. the process of learning through personal experience), and consequently we encourage you to use this approach in your engagement with the book. Although this is not a self-help book and should not be used as a substitute for professional help, often the best way to learn about a particular method is to try using it. So we recommend that you give some thought to what you would like to achieve and to choose aspects of your life you are interested in exploring but which do not represent distressing issues. If your preferred way of learning is more reflective and if you wish to add further understanding to your experiential learning, we have also provided ideas for reading at the end of each chapter.

This book cannot replace the learning that is provided through good-quality training and supervision, but we hope that your interest will be heightened by what you discover in the pages that follow and that you might even wish to develop your knowledge and skills further through undertaking some formal studies. Whatever your reasons for reading this book, however, it is our hope that at the end of it you will have a greater understanding of and appreciation for the work of countless researchers and practitioners who have contributed to the development of this exciting and dynamic field.

Part I

The Principles and Perspectives of Cognitive Behaviour Therapy

ONE

Understanding Cognitive Behaviour Therapy

Chapter objectives

By reading this chapter you will be able to:

- Place CBT in an historical context and understand that it is now a broad-based family of therapies
- Describe the fundamental assumptions that underpin CBT
- Identify common myths and misconceptions about CBT

Introduction

The cognitive behaviour therapies are concerned with exploring the personal meanings, emotions and behaviours that generate or are otherwise implicated in human difficulties. They are concerned with how a person acts (their behaviour), their thoughts, images and the way they process information (cognition), how they feel (emotion) and their physical reactions (physiology). They also take into account a person's history, biological and genetic factors and their current environment.

CBT is a broad discipline, and although united by a common set of foundational assumptions, there are a number of therapies which claim to be cognitive behavioural in focus. This chapter introduces some of these therapies and the foundational assumptions that inform them. It highlights the commitment of CBT to evidence-based practice and challenges some of the common myths that you will encounter when reading critiques of the approach. The overview provided here sets the scene for subsequent chapters which look in depth at some of the specific techniques that arise from these foundational assumptions.

Towards an understanding of CBT

CBT is a family of therapies concerned with helping people change the way they think, feel and act. It has a very wide range of application and can be used to address distressing thoughts and feelings, build new skills to tackle problems, promote well-being and help teams enhance their performance in an organisation – to mention just a few. As is the case with all approaches, CBT does not work for everyone or for all of life's concerns but, when chosen carefully, it is a powerful form of intervention that can increase a person's capacity to survive or even thrive under conditions of adversity. Successful interventions have been demonstrated with children, adults, families, communities and within schools, hospitals and industrial and financial institutions.

First, second and third wave approaches

The different approaches to CBT have sometimes been referred to as first, second or third wave (see Hayes, 2004). First wave approaches are those drawn from the behavioural tradition. This includes the influential work of Pavlov, Watson, Rayner, Jones, Wolpe, and Skinner, the subsequent contribution of Eysenck and Martin (1987) and more recently the work of Spiegler (2015).

Second wave approaches represent the cognitive tradition. This includes the principles and methods derived from the work of A. T. Beck and Ellis, and subsequently the work of J. S. Beck, D. M. Clark, Leahy, Padesky, Persons, and Salkovskis, to name just a few. From classic texts such as Beck et al. (1979) to more recent applications (e.g. CBT for psychosis; see Morrison et al., 2003), this tradition has explored how CBT can be adapted to the needs of an increasingly diverse range of clinical phenomena.

The third wave refers to those approaches which draw upon a range of ideas and create new amalgams of theory to inform practice. Collectively, third wave approaches seek to enhance the effectiveness of the field by capitalising on contextual, functional and experiential strategies of change and through promoting the psychological processes that enable well-being, as opposed to focusing on the reduction of symptoms or the treatment of disorders. Unlike second wave CBT, third wave therapies typically target the processes of thinking rather than specific cognitions. Included in this category of therapies would be mindfulness-based cognitive therapy, compassion focused therapy, acceptance and commitment therapy, dialectical behaviour therapy and metacognitive therapy. These approaches draw upon the work of a wide range of scholars, including Segal, Williams and Teasdale (mindfulness-based approaches), Gilbert (compassion-based approaches), Linehan (dialectical behaviour therapy) and Wells (metacognitive therapy).

Although distinguishing between different waves of CBT has been contested by some (see Hofmann & Asmundson, 2008), for the purposes of this book we find it a helpful device for navigating the rich, diverse and at times conflicting perspectives that inform the field. In particular, and for the purposes of an introductory text, we focus specifically on the first (behavioural) and second (cognitive) traditions as these represent what most would regard as the fundamental underpinnings of the approach.

The historical context of CBT

Behavioural approaches form the first wave of CBT. These have their origins largely within the discipline of experimental psychology and can be traced back to the first psychology department at the University of Leipzig, established in 1879. Here, Wundt developed structured ways to analyse sensory processes, thoughts and reaction times. This early work laid the foundations for creating an understanding of human behaviour through controlled experiments. The main early contributors to what became behavioural therapy lay in the pioneering work of Pavlov and Skinner.

Pavlov's contribution, from the 1890s onwards, lay in the recognition of the role of stimulus in determining behaviour. His most famous experiment involved work with dogs. He discovered that if dogs were presented with food, they will begin to salivate. This is an unconditional stimulus because the effect happens before any learning is introduced. Pavlov demonstrated that if the experimenter took a neutral stimulus (e.g. the sound of a bell) and paired it with the presentation of food, the dogs learned to associate the sound of the bell with food and so began to salivate to the sound of the bell. This was termed the conditional stimulus. Pavlov later found that this response generalised to other features of the environment, such as a dog being led into the experimental laboratory.

Much of human behaviour is also learned through a process of conditioning in which we learn to associate novel stimuli with familiar ones. In the 1920s, Watson and Rayner began to use this understanding to develop research into human patterns of behaviour, such as anxiety responses. They showed how a fear of a neutral object could be conditioned through pairing it with an object that generated fear (such as a loud noise). Correspondingly, during the 1920s Cover Jones (1924, 1926) conducted a series of experiments that demonstrated how such fears could be directly deconditioned by pairing a pleasant stimulus with the feared one to gradually reduce the fear reaction. She later developed a wide range of interventions to deal with fear responses and was also one of the originators of longitudinal studies of childhood which generated considerable interest in child development.

The relationship between stimulus and response, termed classical conditioning, remains central to behavioural approaches to this day. Therapists working within this tradition consider the behaviour of interest and try to identify what stimulus reliably precedes it: that is, the antecedent.

The other main contribution to behavioural approaches lies in understanding the relationship between behaviour and its consequences. This emerged from a variety of sources but principally from the work of Skinner, who demonstrated that behaviour was shaped and maintained by its consequences. For example, rewarding a behaviour increases the likelihood of its being repeated. This process of operant conditioning provided the gateway to numerous studies and applications in fields such as education and therapy. By the 1970s it was used widely to manage violent behaviour, to promote pro-social behaviour in adolescents, in machine-based learning and on patterns of consumer behaviour. As for classical conditioning, the research base for operant conditioning continues to develop (Staddon & Cerutti, 2003).

At the same time as behaviour therapy was growing in popularity, other scholars became interested in cognition – a perspective that was neglected during the rise of behaviourism. This interest has a long history in the field of philosophy. For example, Emmanuel Kant sought to understand how we perceive the world. He made major contributions to our understanding through recognition of features such as the way our perceptions of the world are filtered through our subjective consciousness. Another philosopher who has proved influential on the development of cognitive approaches is the Greek philosopher Epictetus, who argued that, as human beings, we are distressed not by events but by the views which we take of those events. Perhaps, however, the most commonly cited influence on CBT is the Greek philosopher Socrates, who taught his students not by providing them with facts but by asking them a series of questions aimed at uncovering inconsistencies in their thinking. By exposing these inconsistencies, and through the application of critical reasoning and logic, he sought to help his students arrive at more robust and reliable conclusions about life's most pressing concerns (see Chapter 4 for how the Socratic method is used in CBT).

The modern use of earlier philosophical ideas developed from the work of Ellis from the 1950s and Beck from the 1960s. Parallel fields which emerged, such as personal construct psychology (Kelly, 1955), symbolic interactionism (Mead, 1932) and social constructionism (McNamee & Gergen, 1992), explored similar issues in the way our perceptions of the world are co-constructed and shape how we interpret what happens to us. The essence of the cognitive tradition was the need to revisit the question of how behaviour might reflect the way we think about the events that happen to us. Hence, rather than a focus on the stimulus response pattern, cognitive theorists looked at how behaviours were shaped by the beliefs we hold and our perceptions of the world, which inform how we interpret our circumstances and choices. While behavioural and cognitive approaches developed as different traditions, there were, during the 1970s, attempts to combine them. Perhaps the most notable example of this was the work of Meichenbaum, who brought practitioners together to share their ideas on applications of behavioural and cognitive approaches and to explore what each could contribute to the other. He later attempted to synthesise these into an integrated approach (Meichenbaum, 1976). In the UK, the British Association for Behavioural Psychotherapy, founded in 1972, subsequently changed its name in 1992 to incorporate cognitive approaches. As interest in the field grew, research on effectiveness followed and demonstrated the value of CBT as an intervention of choice for a range of difficulties (see Roth & Fonagy, 2005). Thus, the family started as an amalgam of behavioural and cognitive therapies but quickly came to incorporate a range of ideas sharing common assumptions. Theoretical and technical developments in both behaviour therapy and cognitive therapy have continued so that, while the origins remain important, our understanding of concepts such as conditioning has evolved.

CBT as an evidence-based intervention

A claim made by CBT therapists, commissioners and increasingly communicated to clients and other stakeholders is that CBT is evidence-based. Many studies have examined this claim, including Roth and Fonagy (2005) as well as national bodies such as the National Institute of Health and

Care Excellence (NICE, 2004a, 2004b, 2011, 2019). The value of CBT and its potential contribution to enhancing the well-being of the population was recognised in England's 'Increasing Access to Psychological Therapies' (IAPT) initiative (Department of Health, 2008). This has led to a significant expansion of the CBT workforce to deliver treatments for a range of common mental health problems. We discuss this further in Chapter 11.

The empirical evidence underpinning the approach has made a persuasive case for why CBT needs to be more widely accessible. While the evidence for the effectiveness of CBT is strong in some cases, it is not effective for all clients with all conditions and the field is not without its critics (Gaudiano, 2008). Nonetheless, claims for specific therapies conducted under controlled conditions are robust. For example, Hofmann et al.'s (2012) review of meta-analytic studies on the efficacy of CBT concluded that the evidence base is strong, particularly for anxiety disorders, but weaker for other problems. More recently, David et al. (2018) repeated the assertion that CBT is effective but highlighted that there is no room for complacency. However, David et al. (2018) see a positive trend in that CBT is an evolving landscape of practice which is committed to seeking evidence and believe that this may encourage a more research-informed approach among other psychotherapeutic traditions. Nevertheless, there are dissenting voices (Goldiamond, 2002).

Fundamental assumptions that underpin CBT

In its approach to understanding clients' problems, CBT typically differentiates predisposing factors from precipitating and perpetuating factors. In other words, the factors implicated in getting a problem going in the first place are not necessarily those that maintain it. These distinctions are evident in the literature. For example, the relationship between patterns of behaviour difficulty and factors including a person's childhood, community, family, socioeconomic status, gender, health and temperament have long been recognised (Rutter, et al., 1976). In addition, early environmental stress and multiple stressors over a period of time have been shown to increase the likelihood of difficulties in later life (Doom & Gunnar, 2015). However, it cannot be inferred that a difficult childhood *causes* subsequent mental health issues. From a CBT perspective, the exploration focuses on the patterns of belief and behaviour that have been learned as a result of those experiences. An additional focus is the current situation and the identification of factors that maintain specific patterns of cognition and behaviour.

The ABC framework provides one useful way of summarising the enquiry that therapist and client undertake. Of particular interest are events which precipitate a behaviour or emotional response, also known as the antecedent (A) and what follows the behaviour (B), also termed the consequence (C).

The idea of exploring the ABC pattern is common within behavioural and cognitive approaches, although there is a difference of emphasis. Specifically, behaviourally-oriented therapists consider antecedents in terms of stimuli that act as triggers and view consequences as potential reinforcers for the behaviour. Behaviours are those actions that can be directly observed. In contrast, cognitively-oriented therapists, while also concerned with antecedents, are interested in uncovering patterns of thinking and the specific cognitions that they trigger. Consequences are likely to be understood as outcomes of thinking patterns or cognitions. Both orientations explore any protective factors, strengths or opportunities that the client brings or that the context creates that could overcome or mitigate the negative effects. Examples of how predisposing, precipitating, perpetuating and protective factors are considered can be found in the subsequent chapters of this book.

Once the relevant patterns are identified it becomes possible to create a formulation that reflects a theoretically-informed understanding of what is happening to generate the issue of concern (see Chapter 10). Any intervention plan that is subsequently developed will take account of the thoughts, feelings or actions that the client wishes to increase and decrease. At times, the client may be hampered by the absence of a repertoire of skills. This is where CBT has developed a range of approaches, such as social skills training and emotion regulation skills, to instil adaptive behaviours. Discussing with the client what patterns they want to increase, decrease or instil is an empowering way of helping them take control of the change process (Lane, 1978, 1990; Welsh Assembly Government, 2012; Bruch, 2015).

Common myths and misconceptions

As we hope we have demonstrated, CBT is a sophisticated, creative and evolving family of therapies that attempts to be responsive to the needs of those who seek psychological support and the changing needs of our society. Despite variations in perspective and method, what all the approaches share is a commitment to evaluating and refining their effectiveness through use of carefully controlled studies and the development of scientific evidence. Nonetheless, CBT has also attracted myths and misconceptions. Some of the most espoused myths are those that we list below.

1. CBT methods are mechanistic, cold and controlling

While CBT has developed and draws upon a diverse range of techniques to support people in making changes, these are always applied in the context of a warm, supportive and collaborative working relationship. A review of the work of contemporary CBT scholars evidences the emphasis that is placed on the importance of building rapport and creating an effective working alliance. As Meichenbaum (1976), an early developer of CBT, Meyer (see Bruch, 2015), a pioneer of behavioural approaches, and Beck et al. (1979), who pioneered cognitive therapy, have all highlighted, the relationship between therapist and client is central to the work.

2. Cognitive methods are about treating symptoms not the person

CBT is a biopsychosocial approach to intervention; that is, it is concerned with the body, our emotions, the way that we make sense of our worlds and the interpersonal contexts in which people live. There may be times when the agreed focus of therapy is one of targeting a specific mental health disorder (subsequent chapters in this book provide some examples of this), but the notion that CBT is a 'symptom fix' is misplaced. While it was a common assumption among critics in the early days, as CBT has expanded its approach this myth has become less tenable.

3. CBT fits clients to protocols rather than tailoring its approach to the client

It is sometimes claimed that CBT simply applies protocols to disorders rather than being concerned with the client's history, relationships and context. Where they exist, protocols can provide valuable guidance to therapists on what approaches might work best, but these must always be matched to the client. The application of a protocol without due reference to the individual client would not be considered good practice.

4. CBT ignores the client's past and only focuses on the present

The difference between CBT and some other therapeutic modalities is the approach to the past. For the CBT therapist, the past is of interest to the extent that the client's learning history predisposes them to certain patterns of response rather than others. The past is not explored and worked through extensively in order to gain insight, as happens in psychoanalytic methods. However, restructuring problematic aspects of the past happens when therapists work with clients' core belief and schema, or in the context of long-term client issues such as chronic low self-esteem, interpersonal problems and personality disorders. Predisposing factors do, therefore, matter as they help make sense of the person, their history and the contexts in which they have learned how to think, feel and act.

5. The approach takes away the client's agency

CBT is collaborative and works with the client to build a shared understanding of the issues that need to be addressed and a plan to intervene which involves creativity and input from the client. The agency of the client is central to progress and any approach which fails to build on the client's own commitment to change is unlikely to succeed.

6. CBT is limited to the current evidence and so cannot help clients presenting with complex or unique issues

CBT strives to be evidence-based and its practitioners will always seek research to inform the work that they undertake with clients. However, CBT also draws upon experimental, hypothesis-driven approaches. Where there is no comprehensive evidence-base on which to draw, the client and therapist work together to create experiments to explore likely factors of influence that could be modified. In this way complex conditions can be examined and the unique learning history of the client incorporated into the work.

7. CBT is concerned with positive thinking

A particularly common myth is that CBT aims to eliminate negative thinking and help clients 'think positively'. Negative thinking is sometimes an appropriate and adaptive response to the situation in which we find ourselves. If an event occurs which is distressing, the ability to perceive its negative aspects and to experience the negative feelings that go with it are important parts of learning and growing. Negative thoughts can, when adaptive, serve an important self-corrective and at times protective function. Equally, positive thinking – if not tempered by a realistic evaluation of oneself and one's circumstances – can be detrimental. For example, excessive self-belief in a health care professional might result in the assumption that "I'm great at what I do, so I can take short-cuts", resulting in a failure to consider the scientific basis for their decision-making. Unfettered positivity is, therefore, likely to lead to rash decisions, inappropriate risk-taking and poor judgement that has the potential to harm others as well as ourselves.

What therapists are aiming for, then, is *wise* and *flexible* thinking. CBT seeks to empower clients by encouraging them to better understand the way in which they are making sense of the world, identify ways in which their current cognitive stance is proving unhelpful, and broaden their perspective to consider new ways of responding to their circumstances and needs.

Conclusion

CBT is a family of therapies drawn from distinct traditions yet united by a common set of foundational assumptions. Chosen with care it is a powerful form of intervention. Although it is beyond the scope of this chapter to provide more than an introduction to the different therapies within CBT, the main message is that the theory and practice of CBT is a rich, evolving and dynamic terrain in which many ideas are present. These ideas are sometimes seen as being in conflict and sometimes represented as a collaboration but, collectively, they provide many concepts and methods that therapists and clients can draw upon to enable change.

The contexts in which CBT has been applied are highly diverse and include therapy, school-based interventions, parent training, organisational team development and sports science. It is not as is sometimes asserted by its detractors a cold and mechanistic therapy, but rather one based on collaboration which emphasises clients' own agency in bringing about change. As we shall see in subsequent chapters, the application of these ideas and the techniques that they have generated enable clients to become their own therapists to address not just current but also future concerns. This is a sophisticated and long-standing framework for practice.

Reflective Activity: Getting the most from this book

Think about what you most want to gain from reading this book. As you read through each chapter, starting with this one, you might find it helpful to consider your responses to the following questions:

- What did I learn?
- What, if anything, surprised me?
- Were any ideas that I held about CBT confirmed or challenged?
- Having gained an initial sense of the book from this opening chapter, what now is my purpose in reading it? How will I know if that purpose is met?

We recommend that you keep a record of your reflections as you work through the book, noting specifically any ways in which your understanding of CBT changes.

Interested in learning more? Check out ...

Kennerley, H., Kirk, J., & Westbrook, D. (2017). *An introduction to cognitive behaviour Therapy* (3rd ed.). London: SAGE.

TWO

The Cognitive Principle

Chapter objectives

By reading this chapter you will be able to:

- Understand the cognitive principle and why it is central to CBT
- Understand the role that cognition is believed to play in psychological problems
- Explain the difference between cognitive content and cognitive processing
- Identify the different levels of cognition with which CBT therapists work

Introduction

All cognitive behaviour therapies share the view that cognition has a crucial role to play in the development, maintenance and treatment of psychological problems. This foundational assumption lies at the heart of what has been called the 'cognitive principle' in CBT.

In this chapter, we examine what is meant by the term, 'cognitive principle' and how this informs therapists' understanding of and approach to working with clients. We explore what therapists mean when they talk about 'cognition', differentiating cognitive content and processing, as well as different levels of cognition. Readers are also introduced to some of the commonly occurring cognitive biases that can prevent clients from appreciating more helpful perspectives on their circumstances and needs, and that are often a target of subsequent intervention. This chapter provides a foundation for the techniques that are described in Chapters 5–7.

What is meant by the 'cognitive principle'?

Human beings are driven by the need to make meaning out of their experiences. When something happens to us – good or bad – we typically try to understand why it has occurred, what it means about us, others or our life more generally and what implications it has for our future. We locate these events in a bigger mental picture of who we are as individuals, in relation to others and in the context of the lives we lead.

The ways in which clients make sense of their circumstances is deemed critical to understanding their difficulties and needs. It is also elevated to the heart of our attempts to help them create meaningful change. This is known as the cognitive principle.

The cognitive principle states that when an event occurs, we do not simply have an emotional or physical reaction to it; that is, there is no simple, linear cause–effect relationship between an event and how we respond emotionally or physically. As a result, if we say, "When this event occurred, I felt happy/sad/angry…", we are missing a critical piece of the puzzle. In fact, when an event occurs, we interpret what has happened to us and this interpretation is critical in shaping the way we react. If we were going to present this visually, it might look something like Figure 2.1.

The mediating influence of cognition can help us understand why we react to situations and events in the way that we do. Consider, for example, the two individuals described below who are reacting to the same situation in very different ways.

It is important to remember that there is not necessarily one thought for each emotion. Often the situations we encounter give rise to a variety of thoughts and feelings. Also, note how in each scenario both of our

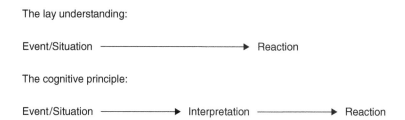

The lay understanding:

Event/Situation ——————————————→ Reaction

The cognitive principle:

Event/Situation ——————→ Interpretation ——————→ Reaction

Figure 2.1.   The cognitive principle

unsuccessful candidates felt bad – given the circumstances, it would have been strange and potentially counter-productive if they had interpreted this outcome in a positive way ("I am a great catch – the organisation was just too stupid to recognise it!"). Nonetheless, each response has profoundly different implications for what the person does next. Person A falls into a pit of hopelessness and despair and becomes disempowered in their search for a new job. Person B allows themselves to hurt – for a while – but approaches what has happened with a mindset that in the longer term is going to enable them to move forward. The mental perspective we take,

---

Situation: Being rejected for a highly desired job after interviewing unsuccessfully for the position.

Person A:

Interpretation: I didn't get the job because I'm useless. I never do well in interviews. I'll never get another job – it's hopeless. Things never work out for me!
Emotions: Shame, embarrassment, hopelessness, sadness
Behavioural responses: Ceases to apply for other jobs, stops looking for new positions, begins to under-perform in current role, withdraws from colleagues.

Person B:

Interpretation: I'm so disappointed – I really thought that this was the job for me. But I obviously didn't manage to convince them that I was a good fit with the company or that I had the right skills. I'm not sure where I fell down so I need to get some feedback and make sure I learn from this for future job applications. It might have just been a very competitive process.
Emotions: Disappointed, anxious but also hopeful
Behavioural responses: Phones up organisation to ask for constructive feedback on interview performance. Organises some interview skills training for future interviews. Continues to search and apply for jobs.

---

according to CBT therapists, can make the difference between staying stuck or moving forward with our lives.

The cognitive principle does not claim that our thinking *causes* emotion in any straightforward, linear way (this would be inaccurate given what we know about emotions from a neuroscience perspective). Rather, cognitive approaches advocate that there is an intimate link between cognition and emotion and believe that one of the most effective ways of facilitating change at the level of emotion is to modify maladaptive patterns of cognition. In order to do this effectively, we need to understand what exactly is meant by 'cognition'.

What is meant by 'cognition' in CBT?

The term 'cognition' is a simple label for a complex array of human experiences that encompass how we perceive the world around us and how we interpret the events that happen to us. Thus, when CBT therapists refer to cognition, they are describing not only the content of a person's cognitions (i.e. what they are thinking) but also their cognitive processing (i.e. how they are perceiving and processing incoming information). Each of these elements is described in greater detail below.

Understanding cognitive content

There are a number of categories of cognition that are of interest to the CBT therapist. These are summarised in Table 2.1.

Table 2.1. Categories of cognitive content in CBT

Thoughts	The voice inside our head that provides an ongoing commentary about the events taking place at any given moment, or about which we are consciously contemplating. Often termed 'automatic thoughts', they can be positive (e.g. "I worked so hard on that report – I'm really pleased with the outcome after all the effort that went into it"), neutral (e.g. "I must remember to pick up a pint of milk on the way home"), or negative ("My boss said she didn't have time to talk to me today as she had to rush off to another meeting. She obviously dislikes me and couldn't wait to get away"). The latter, termed negative automatic thoughts or NATs, are a focus of many cognitive approaches.
Assumptions	Assumptions refer to deeper levels of belief about how things actually are, such as human nature or how the world works. As mental templates that we use to guide us through life, once developed we rarely question them and may not be fully aware of their impact upon us. Like NATs, these can be adaptive (e.g. "If I treat others as I would like to be treated, I'll have good relationships with people most of the time") or negative (e.g. "I must excel all the time otherwise people will find out how incompetent I am and reject me"). The set of assumptions (or rules for living as they are sometimes called) that we develop represent a complex matrix of ideas about how the world works and our role in relation to it, based on our personal history and past experiences. The therapist is likely to look out for those assumptions that appear to be implicated in the area of difficulty for which a client is seeking help, and to work towards developing new, more adaptive rules for living where this is necessary.

Standards	Unlike assumptions which are concerned with how things are, standards are concerned with our beliefs about how things *should* or *must* be (e.g. how people should behave). We can, and typically do, hold standards for ourselves, for other people, for our relationships and for others more generally. When adaptive they create opportunities for personal growth but when excessively demanding they can be problematic. Standards are often expressed in terms such as 'must' and 'should' and CBT therapists are carefully attuned to clients who use these words to describe their experiences.
Attributions	Attributions are the inferences we make about the causes of events. There is probably a good reason in evolutionary terms why we search for causes – when we are successful at figuring things out, it increases the predictability of our world and what is predictable is potentially safer. However, our attributions can prove problematic, especially given that we can sometimes jump to conclusions prematurely and in the absence of adequate evidence. When a therapist asks a client about the evidence they used to arrive at a particular conclusion, they are often seeking information about the client's attributions.
Core beliefs	Unlike assumptions which are conditional ("If A... then B"), core beliefs are fundamental, unconditional beliefs about ourselves, others and how the world works. Often expressed as "I am...", "others are...", "the world is...", many of our core beliefs are developed in the first few years of life as we gauge who we are in relation to those around us. Where a child is fortunate enough to grow up in a home where they feel cared for, respected and where they know they can rely on the grown-ups around them, that child is likely to conclude, "I am safe, loved and capable in the world" and "I can trust people to take care of me". However, if a child grows up in an environment where a parent is erratic in their caregiving, perhaps as a function of their own mental health difficulties, or where there is physical or emotional abuse, they are likely to learn very different things, such as, "I am unsafe, I am unlovable; others are unreliable and can't be trusted; the world is a dangerous place". These fundamental beliefs are believed to provide the templates from which we develop rules for living ("Others aren't trustworthy so the only person I can rely on is me"; "Never let people get too close – if you do, they'll hurt you"; "Avoid conflict at all cost or else you'll get hurt").

Like assumptions and standards, core beliefs can be harder to access as they exert an influence that is often outside conscious awareness. Moreover, because they are developed over time and based on personal experience, the client is likely to assume that "this is just the way life is" and so may not feel inclined to reveal their core beliefs spontaneously. |
| Images | We don't always think in words. Often our cognitions take the form of images – static pictures or mini-movies that occur in the privacy of our minds – that arise instead of or in addition to verbal cognitions. At times this can be entertaining (fantasy often takes the form of imagery) and can be useful (rehearsing a challenging event in our mind in advance of the event itself) but at other times our imagery can be problematic for us. |
| Schemas | *Schemas* refer to a mental framework that helps us organise our experience. Rather like the difference between hardware and software in computing, schemas are the software that enable us to do things in particular ways. Schemas are internal patterns of experience, including emotions, memories, thoughts and beliefs. They are believed to develop in childhood based on the extent to which core needs for love, care and security are met.[1] |

[1] Sometimes in the literature the term 'core belief' is used interchangeably with 'schema', but these are different constructs. A schema refers to complex information-processing structures rather than individual beliefs. Although schema therapies have been developed, they represent specialised applications of CBT and a consideration of these is beyond the scope of an introductory text.

The categories in Table 2.1 refer to what we might term cognitive *content* – that is, the specific form that mental activity takes and upon which people can comment. When a CBT therapist asks the commonly used question "What went through your mind just then?", they are usually asking about content, trying to understand what might lie between the situation in which the client found themselves and their subsequent emotional reaction or behavioural response.

In reality, a client's story often comprises a mix of cognitions at different levels exerting a reciprocal influence. The case of Sandy, a client presenting for help with obsessive-compulsive disorder, provides an example of how these different layers of cognition interacted to escalate her distress and diminish her quality of life and ability to function.

Case study: Sandy

Sandy presented with distressing intrusive cognitions (negative automatic thoughts and images) that featured her stabbing people who were important to her, including her priest, her friends at church and her friends' children for whom she regularly baby-sat. She was adamant that she had never harmed anyone and had absolutely no desire or urge to do so. As a result, the presence of these thoughts and images were highly distressing and she felt at a loss to know why they were occurring (i.e. she could not make an attribution for their presence).

Sandy's intrusive thoughts and images had emerged following a traumatic incident at work in which she had been bullied by a co-worker. Sandy had no sense of why these intrusions had started, but she did reveal that she had always tended to "over-think things". She also believed that she should always look for the best in people as this brought her closer to God (a standard). In her view, "Good people don't have wicked thoughts, so if a person has wicked thoughts it must mean they are a bad person" (assumption).

In terms of her background, her therapist noted that Sandy had grown up in an environment where her father was physically violent towards both her and her mother. She recalled her mother telling her that her father "did these things because he was a bad man", and that "God would punish him for his wickedness".

Because Sandy's thoughts and images were distressing, she made a conscious effort to push them out of her mind (a cognitive strategy known as thought suppression). Yet the harder she tried to suppress the thoughts and images, the stronger they seemed to become. To her this was evidence that "These thoughts are unstoppable" (a negative automatic thought) and "...are powerful and significant" (an attribution about the thoughts and images based on understandable but incomplete information – engaging in thought suppression is known to increase the presence of intrusive thoughts and images). Because she could not suppress her thoughts and because they seemed too dangerous to leave unchallenged,

Sandy would engage in a series of prayers, carried out in a strict order to try to silence the cognitions (a mental ritual designed to neutralise the intrusive thoughts which is also known to increase them). Yet despite her efforts, nothing she attempted seemed to work.

Sandy ceased going to church and stopped praying, as she believed that "God could not love someone who was entertaining such wicked thoughts" (assumption). Because of her cognition that "Good people should not have bad thoughts" (a standard), she concluded that "If I am having bad thoughts, I must be a bad person" (an assumption). She also believed that "Having a thought is as bad as doing the action" and "If I have the thought, I am likely to act on it" (assumptions that also refer to a process known as thought-action fusion, which is common for people experiencing these types of thoughts and images).

Sandy's difficulties illustrate the continual intertwining of a range of levels of cognition, coupled with complex life circumstances – past and present. Although the case study describes a client in distress, it is important to recognise that these levels are believed to be operating for all of us all of the time.

As noted earlier in the chapter, the content of a person's cognitions is only part of the picture. An additional, and equally critical, element is that of cognitive *processing* – how we go about the task of making sense of the world and the situations in which we find ourselves. This is considered next.

Understanding the role of cognitive processing

In any situation we must, of necessity, attend selectively to the information that bombards our senses. Our mental architecture, while highly sophisticated on some levels, is also limited in others and imposes restrictions on the amount of information which we can process at any point in time. This is often for good reason. Imagine, for example, how disruptive it would be for an individual if, on their first date with a potential romantic partner, their cognitive equipment forced them to give equal attention to what their date was saying, how they looked, the waiter's outfit, the conversations between diners on the surrounding tables, the pictures on the walls, the noise of the traffic outside the restaurant, and so on. Attending equally to all of the sources of information that bombard our senses would work against our own best interests – in this case, securing the interest of the prospective romantic partner.

We will always, therefore, be engaged in a process of perceiving and attending to certain types of information at the expense of others and this ability is highly adaptive. Without it we would quickly become overwhelmed

and unable to function – possibly even have our chances of survival threat-
ened if we couldn't selectively attend to signs of danger over neutral and
irrelevant information. Equally, optimal functioning often requires an ability to make short-cuts based on patterns of assumptions that derive from
past experience. Imagine how time-consuming everyday life would be if we
approached daily activities as if we were encountering them for the first time.
We would never get anything done! However, these short-cuts can also bias
our information-processing in ways that are problematic. Table 2.2 lists some
of the most common reasoning biases to which CBT therapists are alert.

Table 2.2.   Common reasoning biases

Type of thinking trap	Description and example
All-or-nothing thinking (also known as dichotomous thinking)	Viewing situations and events from extreme perspectives with no middle ground: e.g. "It was a complete waste of time."
Over-generalising	Drawing sweeping, generalised conclusions: "I've made one mistake on my project, so the whole thing is a disaster."
Catastrophising	Exaggerating the significance of an event. For example: "If I don't achieve my goals, it will be the end of the world."
Mind-reading	Making assumptions about what another person is thinking in the absence of supporting evidence.
Fortune telling	Predicting future events, usually in a catastrophic way, in the absence of supporting evidence.
Discounting positives	Discounting positive information about oneself or the situation and playing down one's strengths and accomplishments.
Exaggerating negatives	Focusing entirely on the negative aspects of a situation and failing to appreciate more positive aspects.
Labelling	Summing oneself up in a single, usually critical or judgemental word: e.g. "I am stupid"; "I am a failure."
Personalising and blame	Blaming ourselves for outcomes for which we are not totally responsible: e.g. "It's my fault my son failed his maths test, because I have been too busy at work lately to help him revise."
Shoulds	Focusing on how things ought to be, often imposing arbitrary rules or standards on oneself or others that become difficult to live up to: e.g. "I should excel in everything I do or else I have failed."
Unfair comparisons	Focusing on others who seem more successful than you (from the outside) and then judging yourself inferior in comparison.
Emotional reasoning	Assuming something is true because it *feels* true: e.g. assuming that you are failing at your job because you feel depressed.

In CBT, therapists are concerned with how the client is processing information about themselves, their circumstances and those around them and
whether these activities are taking place in ways that are likely to increase
distress. This includes what we notice and pay attention to, the way that we

arrive at a particular conclusion (do we weigh up the information carefully or do we jump to conclusions, making swift decisions prematurely) and our ability to recall certain events.

Being aware of cognitive processing is just as important as being aware of cognitive content because some types of client difficulty and psychological disorders are known to be associated with specific changes in how we process information. Engaging in reasoning biases makes it more likely that we misinterpret events and so, therefore, these biases are often a target of therapeutic change.

Conclusion

This chapter has introduced one of the ideas that lies at the heart of CBT – namely, that the way in which we interpret what happens to us is critical in how we react, emotionally, physically and behaviourally, to the world around us and our experience within it. This 'cognitive principle' is simple to state but, as we have seen, the concept of cognition is complex, encompassing many different functions and attributes of the mind, different levels of thinking and different styles of information-processing.

Reflective Activity: Getting to know how your mind works

Spend a few minutes now, sitting quietly in a place where you won't be disturbed, and start by taking a few slow, gentle breaths. As you relax into the moment, begin to notice the activity of the mind. Is it relatively quiet or does it jump around? What sort of ideas go through your mind? Are they mainly positive, neutral or negative? Do they present mainly as verbal statements (thoughts), images, or both? Taking this snapshot of the activity of your mind, what can you learn about the relevance of the cognitive principle to your own life?

Interested in learning more? Check out …

Beck, J. S. (2020). *Cognitive behavior therapy: Basics and beyond* (3rd ed.). New York: Guilford Press.

THREE

The Behavioural Principle

Chapter objectives

By reading this chapter you will be able to:

- Understand the behavioural principle and why this is central to CBT
- Understand the role that context is believed to play in psychological problems
- Explain the role of antecedents, behaviour and consequence in generating and maintaining emotional and behavioural problems
- Identify the different types of intervention that are central to a behavioural approach

Introduction

In addition to an emphasis on cognition, cognitive behaviour therapies share the view that the development and maintenance of psychological problems reflect the influence of patterns of behaviour that, once identified, are an important target for change. This foundational assumption is sometimes termed 'the behavioural principle' in CBT.

In this chapter, we examine what is meant by the 'behavioural principle' and how this informs therapists' understanding of and approach to working with clients' difficulties. We describe what therapists mean when they talk about 'behaviour' and introduce some of the main principles that inform the interventions which therapists subsequently design. In providing a broad overview of the behavioural methods used in practice today, we consider specifically analysis of antecedents, behaviours and consequences, exposure and response prevention, modelling, behavioural experiments and token economies. This chapter provides a foundation for the techniques that are described in Chapters 8 and 9.

What is meant by the 'behavioural principle'?

The behavioural principle in CBT states that behaviour – that is, those actions that we do and do not take – has a critical role to play in our emotional well-being. Traditionally, behavioural approaches have been organised around a process known as functional analysis. Functional analysis is based on the idea that we need to understand the sequence in which behaviour occurs and that the sequence is functionally related: that is, one thing causes another. Using functional analysis, a therapist and client will seek to observe a behaviour of interest and ascertain the sequence and relationship between the different parts of that sequence. The behaviour must be capable of definition in a way that is observable and includes actions as well as measurable internal states, such as those that can be captured with biofeedback devices. Traditionally, behaviourists avoided self-descriptions of internal states such as thoughts and feelings, although clients' self-reports of such states have become incorporated into functional analysis since the emergence of CBT.

There are several challenges involved in arriving at an agreed definition of any behaviour. First, behaviour is complex: the ways in which we act are typically influenced by multiple factors. Even when it appears to be consistent, there are likely to be variations. From the perspective of conducting a functional analysis, these differences matter and provide clues as to factors that are influencing the occurrence. Second, behaviour is dynamic, changing over both short and longer time frames, sometimes over several years.

Understanding how behaviour has changed helps to understand past and current influences.

There is also the question of who is involved in defining a behaviour of interest. It might be an exchange between a therapist and their client or others might be involved, such as a parent, partner, colleague, teacher, social worker or nurse, any of whom might have important observations to offer. In addition to defining the behaviour of concern it is important to understand what alternatives might be available. Not only do therapist and client need to understand which behaviour needs to change but also what the nature of that change should be.

Once a therapist and client have agreed on the behaviour that they wish to observe, they have defined the 'B' needed for an ABC analysis (we introduced the ABC analysis in Chapter 1). It is then possible to introduce a variety of methods of data gathering that might provide clues to the stimulus events that trigger the behaviour in question. Commonly used methods include establishing a series of observations, interviewing the client about recent examples, creating a checklist for collecting information or asking the client to keep a record of the behaviour of interest.

The stimulus event which triggers the behaviour in question is known as the antecedent. The events that immediately follow upon the behaviour in question are referred to as the consequences of the behaviour. With this information, therapist and client can describe the ABC sequence. If therapist and client collect several examples of these sequences it is possible to discover whether there is a consistent pattern in which it can be reliably assumed that A leads to B and is followed by C. The antecedent provides the stimulus to the behaviour which is followed by the consequence which acts as a reward and therefore enhances the chances of the behaviour being repeated. That there is a *functional* relationship is important; a sequence might occur by chance. What the therapist seeks to establish is whether one thing causes another.

Interventions derived from the behavioural principle

Stimulus control

The use of stimulus control as a technique for change requires the identification of three things:

- The stimulus currently controlling the behaviour – the 'wrong' one
- A definition of the appropriate stimulus – the one you want to control the behaviour

- A procedure to bring the behaviour under appropriate stimulus control

Many of our behaviours are under stimulus control and usually the appropriate one. If there are behaviours that we want to change it is worthwhile considering what might be the trigger and how to change this. Any behaviour that seems to be instantaneously triggered (e.g. the moment a person sees, hears or feels something) may well be under stimulus control. For example, a smoker might light up a cigarette when seated with a cup of coffee; the act of drinking coffee triggers the lighting of a cigarette.

Stimulus control procedures can be applied to numerous behaviours where one event triggers another. Consider the example of an exasperated parent who has told their child repeatedly to hang up their coat when they enter the house. The child consistently throws their coat on the floor and only when told to pick it up do they comply. Now consider the behaviour the parent wants to see happen: the child putting the coat on the hook after entering the house. In the description above a therapist will want to understand what event (or stimulus) precedes the behaviour of putting the coat on the hook after entering the house. In this case, the child puts their coat on the hook when told to pick it up off the floor by their parent. In behavioural terms the act of putting the coat on the hook is triggered by being told to do so; that is, the stimulus controlling the behaviour is the act of being told to put the coat on the hook. Yet the appropriate stimulus is the act of opening the door, leading to the coat being taken off, followed by the coat being put on the hook. In this case, the therapist might work with the child to practise going back outside with their coat on and then entering the house, taking off their coat and putting it on the hook.

Reinforcement

When the consequence of a behaviour serves to increase that behaviour (in frequency or intensity) it can be said to reinforce it. Behaviour can be reinforced positively or negatively. Positive reinforcement occurs where the consequence strengthens the behaviour on which it is focused. For example, between life partners, a thank you or smile in response to a compliment increases the likelihood that the act of giving compliments will increase. Likewise, a teacher who responds to a child who asks politely for help increases the chance of a courteous request in future. If the teacher responds only when the child starts whining, then that increases the chances of whining becoming the standard response. Negative reinforcement occurs where a behaviour is strengthened by escape or avoidance of a consequence. For example, if someone's phobic response enables them to avoid exposure to a feared object, then this reinforces the likelihood of the phobic response being repeated. Stimulus control and reinforcement between them represent the most powerful tools in the behavioural repertoire.

Case study: Enrique

Ten-year-old Enrique was referred to a behaviour support team with the statement, "...he is a disturbed child who has always been a problem and causes a great deal of disruption at school. Everything has been tried and we and all the agencies working with him have given up hope that he will change." The allocated practitioner, Mateo, noted that this statement said much about the frustration of those involved but said little about the behaviours themselves. Thus, the starting point was one of identifying the behaviours that were generating such reactions and concerns.

Using the ABC framework, Mateo sought to understand the problematic behaviour (B) so that he could devise observations which would uncover the stimulus or antecedents (A) and consequences (C) precipitating and perpetuating the behaviour. Yet although Enrique's class teacher, Hannah, could provide considerable background information, this took Mateo no closer to understanding the behaviours that Enrique was exhibiting. Hannah stated that she had extreme difficulty in managing Enrique. She had previously taught his siblings, who were also "problematic" and had been referred to specialist placements. Hannah referred to similar concerns from Enrique's social worker and said that he had also seen a psychologist. In a conversation with the Head Teacher, Mateo learned that the school had no idea how to manage Enrique and his mother was no longer prepared to cooperate with the school. Nonetheless, the school had some sympathy for Enrique and did not want to fail with yet another sibling.

Mateo noted that while those responsible for Enrique could provide a great deal of information and were clearly highly frustrated, there was little in the way of information that could be analysed or hypotheses that could be tested. It was important to recognise and respond to the frustration but to work towards clear statements capable of review. Asking for examples of recent critical incidents provided a way to obtain this type of information.

It seemed that Enrique did not respond to teacher instructions and if pressed would shout, run out of the classroom and only return after considerable persuasion. For a while he would settle and, although not following instructions, would work quietly. Largely, Enrique was left to his own devices. This provided Mateo with some information and an exploration of the problem was possible.

It was agreed that Enrique would be observed in class to test the sequence of behaviour described.

The classroom teaching assistant, Tara, was shown how to make and record observations. Those observations were then explored in a conversation after school. Surprise was expressed by all at how often Enrique did in fact work quietly and did not cause difficulties. In addition, two specific incidents were recorded that helped provide a clearer picture. In the first incident, when faced with work he found difficult, he loudly demanded immediate help from the teacher. If Hannah did not respond, Enrique would shout out, "You are useless! You never help me", and then run out of the classroom. Tara would then follow and spend time trying to discover the nature of the problem and persuade him to return to class. In the second incident, when he was struggling with his work Enrique shouted out and Hannah did immediately try to resolve his difficulty. In terms of this limited area of his behaviour, and accepting that there could be other issues, an initial formulation (a topic that we cover in Chapter 10) of the situation was attempted.

Together, Mateo, Hannah and Tara reviewed the data in order to conduct an ABC analysis. They decided to look initially at the second incident, where Enrique loudly demanded immediate attention from his teacher (B). By reviewing the data, they identified that the stimulus (A) was that he was having difficulty completing the task that had been set. The consequence (C) of his having shouted was that he received the support he needed.

The first situation proved somewhat more complicated but the agreed behaviour of concern was shouting and running out of the classroom (B). What preceded that behaviour (A) seemed to be Enrique's not getting the attention to meet his needs. What followed that behaviour and potentially reinforced it was then getting the attention he needed to meet his needs (C).

This formulation and an intervention plan were discussed with Enrique. His mother was asked to be involved but said that she had given up on him and had no wish to participate in any intervention offered. However, Enrique and Hannah had an informative conversation where it transpired that Enrique had no idea what an appropriate behaviour might look like. He did not know how to manage his feelings of frustration or how to alert Hannah that he needed help other than by shouting. He regarded his current way of managing the situation as effective and so was reluctant to change, but he did agree to being taught how to conduct an observation schedule to discover how other children obtained attention from the teacher. When the results were reviewed, Enrique realised that there were a variety of ways to seek help. He agreed to try two of these and keep a record of the results. He and Tara would evaluate the outcome of this experiment and any implications this might have for Enrique's choices.

In the subsequent evaluation, Enrique agreed that he could gain attention when needed in ways other than shouting. To help maintain this new behaviour in the long term all parties agreed that they would regularly review their approach to ensure that Enrique received the help he needed. At this point, his mother asked to be involved and she and Enrique worked on several behaviours at home that they agreed could be changed. At follow-up, Hannah commented, "It is a joy to have Enrique in my class. He is now so helpful, polite and hardworking. I will be sorry to lose him when he goes up next year."

Next, we briefly introduce some additional behavioural approaches that are commonly used in CBT practice.

Exposure and response prevention (ERP)

ERP can appear to be a counter-intuitive approach. During exposure a client is asked to experience events (thoughts feelings, images, objects and situations) that make them anxious or otherwise distressed. They then make a deliberate choice to *not* engage in the usual patterns of unhelpful (potentially avoidant or compulsive) behaviour they usually employ to combat the anxiety. This is the response prevention part. When using this intervention, it is important that the client stays with the anxiety until it decreases. This process of decreasing anxiety is known as habituation. If a client allows themselves to experience anxiety-provoking situations, then initially the level of anxiety will significantly increase and then it starts to decline (see Chapter 8).

Modelling

Modelling arose from approaches in social learning. Bandura (1971) argued that most behaviour is learned through observing others. This provides a guide for subsequent actions where the context is similar. Bandura's work is particularly influential as it created a link between the behavioural work of the period and the role of environmental influences. The use of modelling for dealing with aggressive behaviour, the extinction of avoidant behaviour and the effects of teacher attention in classrooms, were reported as some of the earliest applications of behavioural approaches in natural environments (O'Leary & O'Leary, 1972).

Modelling provides a powerful way of instilling new behaviours and can be compared with the technique of shaping. In a reinforcement schedule, for example, the intended behaviour is rewarded when it occurs in order to increase the occasions when it is used. However, this technique can only be used if the behaviour in question is already in an individual's skill repertoire. If it is not, but at least some part of the skill set is available, behaviour is gradually shaped through a series of approximations. If no element of the required behaviour is present, there is nothing to shape. This is where modelling is particularly powerful as an entire sequence can be learned through imitation.

Behavioural experiments

Behavioural experiments are used extensively in both behavioural and cognitive approaches and we cover these in Part II of the book. Essentially, they are activities planned to take place either within or between sessions where the client tries a behaviour and observes the outcome. They can be used to test the impact of acting in a new way, to practise the use of a skill, to test a prediction and to test beliefs. For example, Lane (1978) asked children to try out a new behaviour they had learned to see if it made a difference to how a teacher or parent reacted to them. Lane and Corrie (2015) also describe a case where an adolescent who had issues with aggression was asked to observe the behaviour of a teacher whom he saw as powerful. The purpose of this observation was to discover how the teacher managed relationships. The belief held by the adolescent – that it is not possible to be powerful without using aggression – was challenged as he saw the teacher exerting control through using listening and engagement.

Behavioural activation

The use of behavioural activation represents a rediscovery of earlier experiments which found that rather than undertake a detailed ABC analysis it was possible to work directly on changing behaviours. The assumption is that if behaviour changes, then the accompanying thoughts and feelings will also change. This idea was widely used in early behavioural work. At an individual level, it was possible to devise a behaviour plan for a client to try new ways of acting in the world. At an interpersonal level, it was possible to agree a contract for how partners react to each other in the context of an intimate relationship. At a system level, the environment could be planned in such a way that makes adaptive behaviour changes more likely.

Behavioural activation is now widely used in the management of a variety of emotional difficulties. Bradbury (2016), for example, provides an illustration of how this approach was applied to a case study of depression, with an emphasis on exploring the life events experienced and the impact they had on the development of the client's psychopathology. The analysis focuses on the impact of the client's behaviour on access to rewards and punishments, not how they influence the development of beliefs, as would be the case in a cognitive approach. We discuss behavioural activation in more detail in Chapter 7.

Token economies and environmental design

Token economies started to appear in hospitals, prisons and schools in the 1960s. They are an extension of contingency management, which is an effective means of organising reinforcements to ensure that they follow desired behaviour. An example might be where, in a classroom setting, a teacher recognises the desired behaviour and ensures that it is rewarded. A parent might apply the same approach to dealing with behaviour difficulties. An interesting use of the idea is found in Premack's Principle, devised originally by David Premack in 1959 but with contemporary relevance. According to Premack's Principle, any behaviour which is frequently engaged in (a high probability response) when it follows a behaviour less frequently demonstrated (a low probability response) increases the likelihood of the low probability response occurring. Thus, a child who prefers to run about will increase sitting still behaviour if it is followed by periods of running about. If applied well, contingency management can greatly increase the occurrence of appropriate behaviours.

As O'Leary and O'Leary contend (1972), a token economy is essentially an organised reinforcement system in which:

1. There needs to be a clear agreement about which behaviours are to be reinforced.
2. A means to make a reward contingent on a behaviour is agreed. For practical reasons this is usually a 'token' which can stand for the promised reward.
3. A set of rules is established governing the exchange of tokens for agreed rewards.

To give one example, in early work applying a token economy system across classrooms and teachers, Lane (1990) used a good report book. The front of the book stated the behaviours that the child had agreed to try to demonstrate in the classroom. Teachers briefly noted at the end of each lesson if the child had displayed the behaviour and added a positive comment if they wished. No negative comments were permitted to differentiate this from the negative style of report books in use in many schools. Every week the comments were reviewed and the relevant reward obtained. Comments were used to discuss the way the programme had progressed and to help the child reflect on what they had learned.

Token economies began to emerge as a noteworthy intervention in the 1960s and by the mid-1970s were in widespread use. They have continued to be applied in work with disabilities and autism, in couple and family therapy, and to develop life skills following serious mental illness. Their current use is reviewed in Kazdin (2012) and Spiegler (2015). Nonetheless, the use of token economies has attracted criticism, especially in institutional settings where token economies have been misused as a form of punitive control by removing tokens earned as a punishment, and through the granting and withholding of basic requirements. Lane (1990) emphasised that they should be used to reinforce not punish and must rely on a contract to which each party (or a responsible guardian) can legitimately consent.

Token economies became one of the inputs to the developing field of environmental design (Krasner, 1980; Zube & Moore, 1991; Demsky & Mack, 2008). The key to the role of environmental design in promoting well-being and mental health is the extent to which systems can be designed to promote resilience. Krasner (1980) outlined the variety of influences that have impacted behavioural approaches to the design of environments in order to develop healthier, more responsive workplaces that can enable well-being and mental health.

Conclusion

This chapter has introduced another of the ideas that lies at the heart of CBT – namely, that how we behave has a key role to play in how we experience the world emotionally and cognitively. This behavioural principle encompasses a range of ideas and approaches, all of which are located within an experimental model; that is, ideas must be tested and examined but always in a way that is transparent to clients and colleagues.

What emerges from the behavioural principle is a variety of methods that have the potential to operate at the individual level (e.g. the use of ERP to support those experiencing phobias or obsessive and compulsive behaviours), at the interpersonal and systems levels (e.g. programmes of contracted contingency management or modelling with couples, families and groups) and at the wider systems level (e.g. the use of token economies and environmental design to enhance responsive behaviour in the context of modifying whole systems).

Of necessity, we have only briefly introduced the core ideas and approaches that are available to inform practice. Further examples will follow throughout the book to deepen your understanding of how cognitive and behavioural principles come together to create powerful interventions.

Reflective Activity: Applying an ABC analysis to your own behaviour

Think about a personal behaviour you might want to change. Keep a diary and carry out an ABC analysis. What did you learn? Do your results point to an intervention at the A, B or C part of the process? What intervention from those discussed in the chapter might work for you? If you were going to take this forward and plan an approach to change, which method described in this chapter might you use and why?

Interested in learning more? Check out ...

Spiegler, M. D. (2015). *Contemporary behaviour therapy* (6th ed.). Boston, MA: Cengage Learning.

FOUR

The Style and Delivery of Cognitive Behaviour Therapy

Chapter objectives

By reading this chapter you will be able to:

- Understand how the style of CBT facilitates the delivery of the cognitive and behavioural principles introduced in Chapters 2 and 3
- Describe the role of collaborative empiricism in enabling client engagement
- Understand the role of structure in therapy and how this can support an empathic, client-focused approach to working
- Explain the role of guided discovery and Socratic questioning in the therapist's approach to facilitating change

Introduction

In the previous chapters, we identified that CBT is not a single therapy but a growing family of diverse approaches that have different perspectives on how best to facilitate change. Despite their differences, what most of these approaches share is a set of common ideas and principles concerning the style of the therapy, the nature of the therapeutic relationship and the ways in which various interventions are delivered. It is these features that would enable an observer to identify that the therapist is delivering CBT as opposed to, say, psychodynamic or humanistic therapy. In this chapter, we identify some of the main features that comprise the way in which CBT is delivered and provide a rationale for their use.

How is CBT delivered?

It is not uncommon to see CBT defined as an active, structured, directive, goal-focused approach (Fenn & Byrne, 2008). Although accurate on a number of levels, this definition can give rise to misconceptions about CBT as being rigid and mechanistic and implemented by a therapist who is concerned with 'correcting' the client's faulty thinking and maladaptive behaviour through 'teaching' them a series of techniques to address the error of their ways! However, this is far from the case. The work that therapists do with their clients relies on a warm, respectful and authentic interpersonal engagement that enables high-quality teamwork. It is both the nature of the relational engagement and its focus on specific areas of concern, goals and objectives that characterise the way in which CBT helps clients make meaningful changes in their lives. In the next section, we introduce some of the principles and approaches that CBT therapists hold in mind when working towards this end.

Collaborative empiricism

In the early stages of therapy, one of the most important tasks facing therapists is building rapport with their clients; the nature of the relationship that develops provides the 'backbone' to any work that therapist and client subsequently do together. This is particularly important because, at times, CBT therapists need to encourage their clients to engage in tasks that feel uncomfortable. For example, it is now widely recognised that where a client holds an extreme and unrealistic fear of a specific object or situation, progress can only be achieved through confronting that fear. Thus, the spider phobic will need to confront spiders, the socially anxious person will need to enter into social situations and the agoraphobic client will need to learn how to leave the sanctuary of the home environment to engage with the outside world. These tasks all require courage and if a client is going to take steps that might initially feel risky, they need to be sure that they are doing so with the support, guidance and genuine care of their therapist.

The way in which the therapist brings together the relational aspects of CBT with the more technical aspects of the approach is through the principle of collaborative empiricism. The term 'collaborative empiricism' was coined by Beck and his colleagues (see Beck et al., 1979) to explain how the therapy is underpinned by a transparent, partnership-based agenda. In this context, collaboration refers to how therapy is organised around a relationship in which two people come together to work towards agreed ends. Each person contributes a specific form of expertise to the process: the therapist brings their knowledge of therapy, of CBT, of the most up-to-date knowledge and evidence, and their clinical experience of what might be helpful based on working with clients with similar difficulties. The client brings their 'expertise by experience'; only they can know for sure what their daily experience looks and feels like and when change starts to occur. It is the synthesising of these two distinct forms of expertise which ensures that therapy can be both evidence-based and tailored to the needs of the individual client.

Of course, most, if not all, therapies claim to be based on a model of partnership, but each has a different way of approaching this endeavour. CBT adopts a transparent agenda and therapists are likely to share explicitly their hunches, hypotheses and ideas and to check their resonance with clients. While the therapist is certainly not given licence to self-disclose at will, they typically work in such a way that possibilities are kept on the table for consideration and testing. Thus, it would not be uncommon for a therapist to say, "I've been thinking about this area of… and had some thoughts about ways we could help you move forward. Would it be helpful if I shared these ideas with you?" The emphasis is on a process of joint discovery.

Accompanying the idea of collaboration is the notion of empiricism. As we identified in Chapter 1, one of the core values underpinning the approach is that our work with clients should be informed by a scientific approach. In the context of therapy, this means that therapists work with their clients to develop and test out hypotheses that are directly relevant to the client's concerns.

Thus, the term 'empiricism' is used to refer to how therapist and client work together to identify and test the validity of those thoughts, assumptions and beliefs that have been identified as implicated in the client's problems, and to experiment with novel perspectives or ways of acting in the world. Because of the cognitive principle introduced in Chapter 2, CBT therapists are wary of taking predictions, attributions, assumptions and beliefs at face value. Instead, clients are encouraged to see cognitions as ideas to be tested. Subject to testing, a client's previous conviction may be identified as totally true, partially accurate or wholly inaccurate and, as such, open up possibilities for change.

Guided discovery and the Socratic method

A central aim of CBT is to help clients make discoveries that have positive implications for how they live their lives. A further stylistic feature that underpins the approach and of the style of learning that it enables is guided discovery.

Guided discovery has been interpreted in the CBT literature in different ways. Regardless of the interpretation used, at the heart of this approach lies an assumption that clients often have the knowledge that they need to bring about positive change in their lives, but during times of difficulty they struggle to access or implement this knowledge. Guided discovery also draws on an assumption that people are most likely to adopt new perspectives on their circumstances and needs and take life-affirming action if they believe that they have arrived at these perspectives themselves (as opposed to being 'told' what to do by a well-meaning therapist!). In consequence, the therapist uses a style of questioning and exploration that can facilitate the client's ownership of any new perspectives or solutions identified.

In her helpful description of guided discovery, Padesky (1993) describes the four elements of guided discovery as follows:

1. Asking informational questions (i.e. what, where, how, when, etc. so that the therapist and client can develop a clear understanding of the situation or event of concern).
2. Empathic listening (so the client knows that they are being heard and understood).
3. Summarising (so that the therapist and client can be sure that the therapist is understanding correctly).
4. Synthesising questions (a particular use of questions and questioning which we explore below).

The last stage of guided discovery that Padesky identifies – that of synthesising questions – links with another characteristic feature of CBT: namely, the use of Socratic questioning. Socratic questioning originates from the Greek philosopher Socrates, who, as we described in Chapter 1, taught his students not by providing them with facts to learn, but by asking them a series of questions in order to expose flaws in their thinking (de Bono, 2006). However, in therapy its use is not to expose flaws in thinking (which may lead to already distressed clients feeling even more vulnerable), but to help a client search for new perspectives that might fit the evidence of their experience more fully or accurately.

The principle of collaborative empiricism is central to guided discovery. Consider, for example, the following scenario where the client, Lukas, who has a diagnosis of panic disorder, has feared that dizziness is a sign of impending seizure. As a responsible practitioner, his therapist, Aileen, has previously sought a medical opinion on her client's well-being and has been reassured that there is no evidence to support Lukas' concerns and that he is in excellent physical health. As a result, Aileen is confident that she has permission to explore with Lukas whether there might be an alternative, non-catastrophic explanation for his powerful physical sensations.

Case study: Lukas

We join the therapy session at the point at which Lukas and Aileen have just carried out an experiment called 'sensation induction'. This is where the therapist and client deliberately evoke the sensations that have proved so frightening for the client to test out whether what the client fears is going to happen actually *does* happen (NB: when conducting experiments of this nature, the therapist should first check that there is nothing in the client's medical history to suggest that sensation induction would be contraindicated).

Aileen: Wow! I know that was a really big deal for you and I'm so pleased that you were willing to bypass your fear, just for a few minutes, to see what would happen if you did something to intentionally make yourself dizzy. And we agreed that I would do it with you, so we could compare experiences. But, before we talk about what we've just done together, tell me, how are you feeling now?

Lukas: Dizzy! And a bit relieved that it's over (laughs).

Aileen: (also laughs) I got pretty dizzy when we did that, too. And for me certainly, it's not a comfortable feeling. How about for you?

Lukas: I don't like the feeling, either.

Aileen: So, we are agreed – it's not pleasant to feel dizzy, as we've both just discovered. But unpleasant doesn't necessarily mean dangerous and that's what we've been trying to test out. So let's look at what we can learn from what we've just done. Let's start by recapping on why we decided to do this. Do you want to remind us both?

Lukas: To find out whether, when I get dizzy, I really will have a seizure or whether my panic attacks aren't dangerous at all.

Aileen: You've got it. You have been living with the fear that dizziness was a sign that you were about to have a seizure. When we first discussed this, you said that you had absolutely no doubt that this would happen – that you believed it to be 100% true. In fact, you have been so convinced that it's true, you have organised your life around trying to avoid feeling dizzy. At the same time, you've told me that despite your best efforts, there have been several occasions when you became dizzy and that nothing happened. The feelings eventually went away without you having a seizure. It's been difficult for you to make sense of these conflicting experiences. On the one hand, you have been having these strong, unpleasant physical sensations, but on the other, you have never actually had a seizure, your doctors have reassured you that you are fit and well and you have even had occasions when you have become dizzy but nothing bad has happened ...

Lukas: (thoughtful) ... and there is also the information you gave me about panic attacks ... I hadn't realised panic attacks could make you feel so out of control ...

Aileen: Right. So, we came up with these two contrasting ideas, didn't we? The first is that getting dizzy is a sign that you are about to have a seizure. The second is that these sensations are unpleasant but that they are benign – they are not a sign that you are about to have a seizure.

Lukas: Yeah. And if I could find out which one was true it could really help me.

Aileen: Absolutely. Now, we have just spent the last few minutes intentionally making ourselves dizzy by standing up and spinning round and round, and although we both felt very dizzy neither of us has had a seizure. I'm wondering what you make of this, what we might conclude from this experience. What are your thoughts now about whether dizziness leads to seizures? How does this idea fit with the experience you have just had?

At this point, note that Aileen is not trying to convince Lukas of anything. Her role is not to challenge or dispute ("Given that you have been dizzy on so many occasions in the past and have never had a seizure, why haven't you considered the possibility that your idea is just plain wrong?"). Rather, she is trying to create a scenario where Lukas has the opportunity to put to the test his catastrophic fear about the consequences of getting dizzy. Here we can see an example of the collaborative working relationship that we previously identified as so essential to CBT. Without a close and trusting working relationship, this type of experiment is impossible to carry out in a way that feels safe and empowering for the client. While the therapist is likely to be instrumental in suggesting ways in which certain thoughts, beliefs and predictions might be tested, it is ultimately the decision of the client whether to proceed. Interventions are always approached in the spirit of collaboration rather than coercion, with the therapist attending to matters of pacing and timing and never losing sight of the fact that in doing so the client is often demonstrating considerable courage. We examine these types of experiment further in Chapter 9 so you can gain further insight into how these important interventions can be optimally impactful.

At the heart of guided discovery and Socratic questioning is a belief that we all arrive at certain conclusions for good reasons. As we identified in Chapter 1, one of the most common misunderstandings of CBT is that the aim is to think logically or even think positively. In fact, clients often berate themselves for 'failing to think logically'. But in our experience, logic is not the problem. Thus, the style of therapy supports clients in developing an empathic understanding of why they might have come to view a particular situation in a particular way while also identifying how their perspectives might be inaccurate or unhelpful.

One final point to note about Socratic questioning is that it relies upon the client having the knowledge to answer the questions that will help them make the connections. It will not prove helpful if a client doesn't have the knowledge to begin with. At times, the therapist will need to provide supplemental information, such as psychoeducation on the symptoms and effects of different disorders or areas of difficulty, to help the client update their understanding with appropriate knowledge drawn from the science of the discipline.

Use of structure and active practice to guide the journey

By now we hope that we have conveyed that CBT is an approach to working with clients that is grounded within a warm, caring, engaged working relationship – one that is seeking to foster curiosity and create opportunities for learning and discovery. A final element of the style and delivery of CBT is the use of structure and how the approach capitalises on tasks that the client agrees to progress between meetings.

CBT is typically described as a structured approach but the use of structure does not mean that the therapist works rigidly, doggedly going through item after item. Rather, it provides a framework for the session that supports therapist and client in having a shared responsibility for organising and prioritising topics that are of optimal concern for the client. A typical session might involve the following components:

1. Beginning with a brief, initial 'check in' so that the therapist can gain a sense of how things have been for the client since the last meeting (including any major or unexpected events).
2. Obtaining feedback from the client about the last session: what they recall, what was most helpful and anything that was not helpful.
3. Reviewing the client's efforts at active practice tasks between sessions: what worked well or not so well, what has been learned that might be useful for the client's well-being or that might need further discussion in the current meeting.
4. Agreeing an agenda for the meeting that takes account of the agreed priorities.
5. Addressing the priorities for the session (which will usually take up most of the session).
6. Agreeing new active practice tasks to take away and try.
7. Summarising the main areas discussed in the session.
8. Asking the client for feedback on the session.

Active practice tasks are an important ingredient of CBT sessions. No matter how important the conversations are that take place within the consulting room, it is in their daily lives that clients want to see change. Moreover, as therapist and client have only one hour together of the 168 hours that make up the entire week, the work that takes place in the sessions needs to be complemented and augmented by active practice between the sessions if the client is to achieve their objectives.

A second principle that informs the need for active practice is experiential learning (or learning through experience). Learning that is grounded in the evidence of our own experience is generally more persuasive and motivating than passive learning (what others tell us we should do). This links back to the idea of guided discovery, where we identified that the role of the therapist is not to challenge or dispute but rather to think creatively with the client about setting up opportunities for trying things differently in order to obtain information that is critical to them.

A third rationale for the use of active practice tasks is that it promotes a sense of self-efficacy. Discovering that we can do things differently and change how we experience aspects of our lives can build self-confidence in its own right. Without discussing this directly in therapy, a client can learn that they are able to influence and direct their lives in ways that perhaps they had not anticipated, which can promote a sense of resilience and empowerment.

Active practice between sessions can take a variety of forms, but the aim is always to ensure that it is tailored specifically to the needs of the client at a particular stage of therapy. They might be as focused as the therapist providing some self-help materials for the client to read or as fluid as asking the client to notice when things are generally working better and to do more of what seems to enable this. They might include self-monitoring tasks or engaging in specific experiments in changing behaviour in order to observe the consequences. What is important is that the client understands that all of these tasks are in the service of discovery. Where possible, the client sets their own tasks. For example, the therapist might ask: "Based on what we've discussed today, what thoughts do you have about what you'd like to work on in the week ahead?" At times the therapist may offer ideas. Here the therapist might ask: "Would it be helpful if I shared some thoughts about things to take away and try?" Whatever the approach adopted, the more creative the therapist and client can be, the more likely they are to identify meaningful and illuminating tasks that can support the client's efforts at change.

Conclusion

The stylistic features discussed in this chapter provide a set of principles rather than rigid and dogmatic criteria to which therapists need to conform. The ways in which these principles are enacted within any therapy setting will be as idiosyncratic as the therapists and clients who enact them.

Among other considerations, the therapist will need to reflect on the type of interpersonal style that is most likely to enable a particular client to feel safe and flourish in the therapeutic setting. For example, being explicitly warm and using high levels of eye contact may work well for a client with high levels of generalised anxiety but be experienced as aversive for a client with social anxiety disorder. Likewise, a client who has a history of early sexual abuse might view interpersonal warmth with suspicion, associating it with an impending threat (e.g. historically, their abuser was very 'nice' to the client by giving them treats or gifts, or paying them compliments immediately before assaulting them). Some clients prefer a more direct style ("Spare me the touchy feely stuff and tell it to me straight") whereas others may be highly sensitive to signs of criticism, rejection or abandonment (real or imagined) and need more explicit evidence of warmth, caring and concern to feel secure in their therapy.

Regardless of how the stylistic features of CBT are enacted in therapy, collectively they provide the foundations for the variety of specific methods and techniques that comprise the CBT approach. These are examined in Part II of the book.

Reflective Activity: Reflecting on the experience of a change in perspective

Recall a time when you believed something to be true but were later presented with information that led you to revise your belief. Then consider:

- What was the nature of the information that persuaded you to change your belief?
- Did your belief change immediately or over time, through the accumulating of further evidence?
- Was it based on the persuasive argument of another or grounded in your own experience?

Reflect upon your answers and see what clues your own experience might give you about how easy (or difficult!) it can be for us to change our beliefs and the kinds of experiences that enable us to do so, when this is necessary.

Interested in learning more? Check out …

Beck, A. T., Rush, A. J., Shaw, B. F., & Emery, G. (1979). *Cognitive therapy of depression.* New York: Guilford Press.

Part II
Cognitive and Behavioural Interventions

FIVE

Cognitive Techniques for Working with Thoughts

Chapter objectives

By reading this chapter you will be able to:

- Understand the rationale for targeting thoughts in CBT
- Describe the characteristics of automatic thoughts
- Explain how modifying automatic thoughts enables emotion and behaviour-based change
- Describe the cognitive interventions commonly used to modify negative automatic thoughts

Introduction

CBT seeks to access and modify cognitions that are inaccurate, unhelpful or that otherwise interfere with clients' ability to achieve their objectives. There are, then, compelling reasons why a CBT therapist will want to work with thoughts:

1. Working with thoughts is consistent with the cognitive principle that lies at the heart of the CBT model.
2. Thoughts are typically easier to modify than emotions and so working directly with cognitions provides a swifter route to change than targeting emotions.
3. Unhelpful thoughts exacerbate distress and difficulty and so represent a good focus of intervention.
4. Unhelpful thoughts distort our perspective through commonly occurring reasoning biases and we can correct these reasoning biases.
5. Unhelpful cognitions hamper effective problem-solving. When facing difficulties, we need to be able to make sound choices about our situation and needs, which relies on having a clear and accurate perspective on our choices.

As described in Chapter 2, cognitions can take several forms and exist at different levels, some of which are more immediately accessible to conscious awareness than others. In this chapter, we examine those cognitions of which we can most easily and directly become aware: namely, our thoughts.

Negative automatic thoughts

The types of thought that are of concern in CBT are typically referred to as 'automatic thoughts' which accompany us throughout everyday life and have the following characteristics:

1. They occur spontaneously: we do not need to focus effort on uncovering them.
2. They are situation-specific: although we may have similar kinds of automatic thoughts in similar situations, they arise in the context of particular situations or events.
3. They are fleeting.
4. When their content is emotive, they have an immediate effect on how we feel emotionally and physically.
5. They are so much a part of our everyday experience that we tend not to notice when they are present.
6. When we do recognise that they are present, we tend to take them at face value as they seem credible to us.

Automatic thoughts can be positive, emotionally neutral, negative or unhelpful but those of particular interest to CBT therapists are the automatic thoughts that are tied to the difficulties for which a client is seeking help. These are typically negatively oriented and unhelpful – either because they are biased in some way or because they limit a person's ability to appreciate the options available to them.

Negative automatic thoughts (NATs) can take many forms but the theory and research that underpins CBT has shed light on some of the cognitive profiles that are linked to specific presenting problems. Being aware of these cognitive profiles can be helpful in guiding the process of exploration and in illuminating the types of NATs that therapy may need to address. Table 5.1 identifies some examples of the NATS associated with common presenting problems.

Table 5.1. Negative automatic thoughts associated with common client problems

Problem	Negative automatic thoughts
Panic disorder:	Focus of NATs: a catastrophic misinterpretation of a benign physical sensation (immediate consequence anticipated): • I am having a heart attack • I am having/about to have a seizure • I am having a stroke • I am going mad • I am about to die
Illness anxiety disorder:	Focus of NATs: a catastrophic misinterpretation of a benign physical sensation or body state (longer-term consequence anticipated): • A mark has appeared on my skin – I must have cancer • I keep getting headaches. I have a brain tumour. I'm going to die and my children won't cope without me
Generalised anxiety disorder:	Focus of NATs: intolerance of uncertainty often characterised by 'what if' statements: • What if I make a mess of my job interview? • What if my child is in an accident? • What if I lose my job? I won't be able to pay my bills, my children will be taken away, my wife will leave me ...
Obsessive compulsive disorder:	Focus of NATs: a preoccupation with harm and needing to prevent it, as well as a perceived responsibility for preventing harm to self or others: • If I don't check that I locked the front door, I might have left it open, then we'll get burgled and it will be my fault • I can't remember whether I turned off the lights before I went to bed – there could be a fire • I might have driven into a pedestrian when I drove down our street just now – I need to go back and check • I need to keep washing my hands until they feel clean, otherwise they will be contaminated

(Continued)

Table 5.1.   (Continued)

Problem	Negative automatic thoughts
Depression:	Focus of NATs: commonly referred to as the negative cognitive triad involving negative appraisals of the self, the world/life and the future: • I am useless/I am a failure (self) • Everything always goes wrong (life) • The world is a terrible place (life) • The future is bleak (future) • Nothing I do will make things better (future)
Social anxiety:	Focus of NATs: fear of negative evaluation by others: • They will think I am stupid (prediction) • They think I am boring (while in the situation) • He looked at his watch when I was talking to him – he was anxious to get away from me (post-event evaluation)
Anger:	Focus of NATs: the injustice or unfairness of the actions of others, or having one's rules broken: • She is taking advantage of me • They should treat me with more respect • I deserve better • He is trying to undermine me

Thus, although automatic thoughts are a normal and natural part of our cognitive equipment, where they are unhelpful, they are a target of intervention.

Knowing how to identify and help clients modify their NATs is the focus of the next section.

Techniques for working with cognitions

With a little support and some practice, most of us can learn to identify our thoughts, monitor them in terms of their presence, frequency and impact, and revise them in light of new information. In order to help clients to achieve this, CBT has developed a wide variety of techniques upon which therapists can draw.

Methods for eliciting thoughts

Prior to learning how to change them, clients first need to know how to recognise when NATS are occurring. It is not unusual for clients to struggle with this initially – in our everyday lives we tend not to pay close attention to the details of individual thoughts, differentiate them from feelings or attempt to capture them 'in action' in the way that CBT seeks to achieve. As a result, it is important for clients not to feel disheartened if they experience some difficulty with this task, at least to begin with.

The approach to eliciting thoughts that the therapist adopts will depend on the client's needs and the extent to which they resonate with the idea of a link between thoughts and feelings. It is also important for the therapist and client to agree on what would be the most useful information to collect.

Sometimes, it can be sufficient in the early stages to ask a client to simply keep a record of the frequency of specific NATs. Alternatively, the focus might be on identifying moments when there is a change in the client's mood (e.g. sadness) or state of emotional arousal (e.g. anxiety or anger). It may be preferable for certain clients to work on capturing the thoughts associated with a maladaptive urge (e.g. the urge to engage in hand-washing for a client with OCD, or to have a drink for someone who is alcohol dependent). Another common focus is the NATs that occur when a client enters situations that are triggers for emotional difficulty (e.g. social situations) or specific times of day when a target problem is experienced (e.g. first thing in the morning).

There are several questions that the therapist can ask to help a client identify the NATs that are implicated in a situation or event that is distressing to them. These include:

- What was going through your mind just before you started to feel this way?
- How much did you believe this thought at the time (0–100%)?
- What do you think this situation says about you? Other people? Your life? The world at large?
- What is the worst thing that could happen (assuming that this thought is true)?

It is usually advisable to make a note of any NATs as soon after the event as possible as this will make any recordings more accurate and, therefore, useful. Figure 5.1 below illustrates the type of information that a client might capture with a thought record, drawing on the case example of Abdul.

Methods for testing thoughts

Regardless of the method used, the broad aim is to help clients appreciate that their thoughts are ideas to be taken for the testing, rather than statements they can assume are factually correct. As a result, working with NATs nearly always involves helping the client engage in a process of evidence-gathering. Evidence-gathering can take several forms. Often this occurs in the therapy session itself through a process of guided discovery (see Chapter 4 for an example). Kennerley et al. (2017) cite four categories of questions that can pave the way for discovering new perspectives.

1. Questions aimed at eliciting the evidence for the target thought

These questions help the client to appreciate that there is a good reason why they might have arrived at a particular view of a situation. They are an important foundation for building up a more balanced perspective. The types of question that fall into this category include:

- What factors are leading you to conclude that your thought is true?
- What evidence is there that supports this perspective?
- What evidence do you have that confirms your understanding is correct?
- What experiences have you had that suggest this thought is true?

2. Questions aimed at eliciting the evidence against the target thought

These questions are concerned with unearthing any information, experiences, facts or evidence that are not wholly consistent with the NAT and which, therefore, gently challenge or hint at alternative ways of viewing the situation. The types of question that fall into this category include:

- To what extent does your current thought seem to fit the available evidence completely or are there gaps or inconsistencies?
- What evidence might there be to suggest that this thought may not be wholly accurate/the whole story?
- Is there anything in how you are viewing the situation that doesn't quite fit? Are there any small things that you might be overlooking or discounting?
- Have there been any exceptions? Have there been times in your life when that thought has not seemed to apply?
- When you are not feeling distressed in the way that you are at the moment, do you think about this situation in a different way? If so, how?
- Is there any other evidence that we need to take into account here?

When creating a balanced case for the target thought, it is also important to consider the quality of the evidence the client is using to infer their conclusions.

3. Questions aimed at eliciting alternative perspectives

Using the evidence that has been compiled for and against the target thought, it then becomes easier to identify alternative perspectives that may be more helpful for the client. The types of question that fall into this category include:

- How might someone else view that situation?
- What other ways of looking at this situation are there?
- If someone you cared about found themselves in this situation, how would you view things then? What advice might you give them?
- How would someone who cares about you and whose judgement you trust encourage you to think about this situation?
- Based on the evidence for and against the original idea that you had, what other possibilities now strike you?
- How would you need to view this situation for it to become less distressing?
- Based on weighing up the evidence for and against this target thought, does an alternative perspective provide a better, more accurate or more helpful perspective?

4. Questions aimed at eliciting the consequences of holding a specific thought (or its alternative)

Questions concerned with eliciting the consequences of a cognition can help a client appreciate how holding a particular thought benefits or works against their life choices. This can support a more detailed 'cost–benefit' analysis and potentially increase the client's willingness to consider changing their perspective and subsequent behaviour. The types of question that fall into this category include:

- How does this thought impact you? Your life? Your difficulties? The choices available to you in this situation?
- In what way does holding this thought help you?
- In what way does holding this thought work against you?
- What are the consequences of reacting as though this thought were true?
- If your original idea is true, what then are your options?

Case study: Abdul

Abdul was a 50-year-old man who was adjusting to life following a serious road traffic accident that had left him with chronic back pain and mobility difficulties. Following a financial settlement, a period of physical rehabilitation and psychological treatment for pain management, he had recently returned to work.

Abdul had enjoyed a long-standing career in financial services but his return to work was proving challenging. He was particularly concerned about being perceived as weak and "not pulling his weight" and believed that his line manager was seeking to have him transferred to another team. These preoccupations were contributing to an emerging depression and so his employer's Occupational Health Service had referred him for help with low mood and adjustment. Following a period of assessment, Abdul began working with CBT therapist, Stefan.

Abdul responded well to Stefan's explanation of the role of NATs in low mood and they also explored how Abdul's NATs could be influencing his perception of his manager's intentions towards him. Having worked through some examples with Stefan in the session, Abdul agreed to keep a thought record for homework to learn more about the relationship between his thoughts and feelings.

Date & Time	Situation	Emotion/s	Thoughts
	Where were you? What were you doing? Who were you with?	What emotion/s were you feeling? How strongly did you feel each one (0–100%)	What went through your mind? How much did you believe this to be true (0–100%)?
Sunday, 5pm	Sitting in the garden by myself. Began to think about going back to work on Monday. Began playing over in my mind the conversation I had had with my line manager on Friday about how he wanted me to work with a colleague on a new case rather than handle it by myself	anxious (70%) sad (40%) hopeless (80%) angry (60%)	My line manager thinks I am weak and useless and wants to get rid of me (90%) If I make a mistake, my line manager will use it against me (90%) I'll probably end up losing my job (85%) I used to make a difference in my job. Now everyone sees me as a burden (90%)

Figure 5.1.   Abdul's thought diary for eliciting NATs

On reviewing his thought records, and with the help of Stefan, Abdul appreciated that there were several reasoning biases present in his NATs and that he was making many unsubstantiated assumptions. In choosing one specific NAT to work on, Abdul selected the thought, "My line manager thinks I am weak and useless and wants to get rid of me", which he believed 90%. By working through the evidence-gathering questions above, Abdul recognised that he did not really have any evidence for this thought but there was some compelling evidence against it. For example, Abdul's line manager had:

- A good reputation among his direct reports for being a fair-minded and supportive manager
- Repeatedly said that he was committed to helping Abdul return to work
- Encouraged Abdul to speak to him if he was ever experiencing difficulties
- Suggested regular meetings to review his workload and check how he was managing
- Followed the return to work plan agreed with Occupational Health and Human Resources carefully to ensure that Abdul's best interests were served

On balance, Abdul believed that his original NAT was not accurate and, in taking account of both the evidence for and against his original idea, he arrived at a new perspective: "My line manager has consistently demonstrated that he wants to support my return to work. Although I don't know what he has planned for the future, I have no evidence to suggest that he wants to get rid of me." Abdul believed this 80%.

Abdul also recognised that some of his NATs were probably based on his own insecurities about returning to work and whether he could still perform his job effectively. This fear had been exacerbated by his manager instructing Abdul to co-work a new case rather than operate independently as he would have done before his accident. He recognised that because of the assumptions he was making, he was not actually clear about his line manager's reasons for this instruction and so decided to raise this at their next scheduled meeting. Now clearer about his course of action, Abdul's sense of hopelessness – the feeling he had most wanted to change – had reduced from 80% to 20%.

Common pitfalls and how to address them

Working with thoughts seems simple but in practice can pose a number of challenges for therapist and client. When identifying, testing and modifying NATs, the precise nature of the evidence-gathering process used will vary as a function of the nature of the client's needs, their style of learning and communication, and the interaction that unfolds in the context of a therapy session. There are, however, several common pitfalls of which to be aware.

Problems with identifying thoughts

When clients are learning this skill, it is often easier to identify the relevant NATs when the emotion is hot (i.e. present) rather than cold (absent). For example, a client is much more likely to be able to identify their catastrophic prediction of what is about to occur when they are having a panic attack as opposed to when they have been free from panic attacks for six months. Immediacy of experience makes the content more accessible, which is another reason why clients are encouraged to monitor their thoughts for homework.

Problems accessing NAT

At times, a client can struggle to access thoughts. Sometimes this is simply a matter of practice; like all skills, identifying NATs takes time to master. Sometimes difficulties with accessing NATs is a sign that the therapist needs to change their language. For example, our 'thoughts' can take the form of images or movie clips in our minds rather than verbal statements (see Chapter 9). Rather than asking a client, "What did you think in that moment?", which directs them to looking for a verbal statement, it is often preferable to ask, "What went through your mind?", which invites them to search across thoughts and images.

Discomfort arising from identifying NATS

Discovering what our minds get up to can be unsettling. In Western culture we are encouraged to have great faith in our mental capabilities. As a result, it can feel troubling to discover that our minds are not always as accurate in the conclusions they reach as we might have thought. Some clients can even begin to catastrophise about their NATs ("I knew things were bad but now I've discovered I can't even trust how I think! Am I capable of making any decisions about anything?"). It is important to prepare clients for this, especially as they will spend time learning how to identify and monitor their NATs before learning how to change them. Encouraging clients to avoid thinking about their thinking in all-or-nothing terms (see Chapter 2) can also be helpful.

Problems with modifying NATS

Sometimes clients come up with logical alternatives to their NATs which are intellectually appealing but which have no emotional impact. Where this occurs, the client can experience a 'head–heart lag' ("I understand the situation *intellectually*, but it doesn't *feel* true"). Thinking logically is only a part of the picture and rarely emotionally persuasive. The aim is not, therefore, changing thoughts for its own sake, but changing them because new perspectives open up possibilities for the client's lived experience. If a client does not experience any emotional change at the end of the process, it is important to explore why the original thought still feels compelling. Doubts may reflect the presence of further NATs that need exploring; there may be an even 'hotter' thought that is driving the client's distress or difficulty. Alternatively, the client may be engaging in the futile task of trying to challenge facts.

Challenging facts rather than thoughts

Therapists need to make sure that they work to modify NATs, not facts. For example, if a therapist asks a client who has just been made redundant what was going through her mind when she noticed feeling sad and worried, she might say, "I've lost my job". As a statement of fact, it is not possible to look for evidence for and against this thought or to arrive at an alternative explanation of events. Rather, in such a situation the therapist would want to ask a series of additional questions aimed at uncovering the deeper meanings of this event, especially if the sadness and anxiety were intense and potentially emotionally paralysing for the client. Questions that a therapist could ask in this situation might include:

- I can quite appreciate why you would be feeling sad and worried in this situation; being made redundant is a big deal for anyone. When you think about what's happened, what aspects of the situation distress you most?
- What's the worst-case scenario that you have running through your mind? ... and if that did occur, what would happen then? ... and then?
- What do you think that this situation says about you, your abilities as a professional, your future?

The process described above is often referred to as 'downward arrowing'. As part of a process of guided discovery, downward arrowing can help therapist and client uncover NATs or more deeply-held cognitions that are implicated in the client's emotional reaction and illuminate where reasoning biases may be operating. We explore both downward arrowing and deeply-held cognitions in Chapter 6.

Working with questions rather than thoughts

As illustrated in Table 5.1, unhelpful thoughts sometimes take the form of questions rather than statements. A typical example would be the 'what if?' question ("What if I make a fool of myself?"; "What if I lose my job?"). Another common question is the 'why' (e.g. "Why did I mess up so badly?"; "Why am I such a loser?"). It is not possible to search for evidence for and against a question and so where this occurs the therapist will work with the client to change this into a statement. The easiest way to do this is to ask the client to answer the question. This typically uncovers the NAT of concern. For example, answering the question "What if I lose my job?" might lead to, "If I lost my job, I would get behind on my mortgage payments and then we would lose our home. I wouldn't be able to take care of my family and my children would be taken into care…". These latter statements reveal something important about the meaning of the situation to the client and provide a basis for evidence-gathering and the search for new perspectives that might support effective problem-solving.

Conclusion

In this chapter, we have introduced some of the main methods that CBT therapists use to help clients re-examine and, where appropriate, modify their NATs. We have also considered some of the methods and techniques for working with thoughts and some of the challenges that can arise.

As we have emphasised elsewhere in this book, it is important to help clients appreciate that the aim is not to eliminate negative thoughts and promote positive thinking. Negative thinking can be very helpful when it reflects the realities of the situation and promotes effective problem-solving. Equally, positive thinking can be destructive if not tempered by a clear perspective on the situation. The aim is to help clients increase their choices by broadening the cognitive landscape that they have available to them. A useful test of any intervention aimed at the level of NATs is not only does the client feel differently at the end of the process, but how they conceptualise their options. Your goal as the therapist is not to disprove a cognition but to create a gateway to new perspectives.

For many clients, working at the level of thoughts is sufficient. The use of the techniques and methods described in this chapter, often combined with the behavioural methods we explore in Chapters 8 and 9, are what is needed to help the client achieve their objectives. However, sometimes this is not enough and methods are needed to dig a little deeper into a client's cognitive world. This takes us into the realms of working with enduring cognitions, such as assumptions and beliefs, which is the topic of the next chapter.

Reflective Activity: Getting to know your NATs

We all experience NATs from time to time and so it is useful to practise identifying these. Think of a situation where you have a moderately strong emotional reaction and where you would like something to be different in some way. Using a thought record of your own, see if you can identify the NATs that are associated with your reaction. Use the following headings to organise your exploration:

1. Situation
2. Emotion (if several, pick the one that is most upsetting or that you most want to change)
3. Thoughts (if several, pick the one that seems most salient to the situation)
4. Evidence for the hot thought
5. Evidence against the hot thought
6. Alternative and balanced perspective
7. Re-rate the emotion that you identified as most wanting to change

See whether you think or feel about the situation any differently now, having gone through this process.

Interested in learning more? Check out ...

Greenberger, D., & Padesky, C. A. (2015). *Mind over mood* (2nd ed.). New York: Guilford Press.

SIX

Cognitive Techniques for Working with Enduring Cognitions

Chapter objectives

By reading this chapter you will be able to:

- Understand the nature and characteristics of enduring cognitions as conceptualised within CBT
- Describe a range of cognitive interventions aimed at identifying and, where necessary, modifying these deeper levels of belief
- Describe when and how these interventions might be applied in therapy

Introduction

In the previous chapter, we examined ways of identifying and modifying negative automatic thoughts – those situation-specific cognitions that are relatively available to conscious introspection and that tend to fuel a person's distress and unhelpful reactions in the moment. However, our NATs are only part of the cognitive picture. The way that we make sense of the world around us also relies on deeper levels of cognition that shape our lives in more subtle and complex ways.

In this chapter, we examine those more enduring cognitions which are relevant to understanding and working with clients' difficulties. In particular, we focus on conditional beliefs, such as standards, assumptions and rules for living, and unconditional, core beliefs.

The characteristics of enduring cognitions

The enduring cognitions of interest to CBT therapists are those which reflect an individual's deeply-held beliefs about the self, other people and the world around them. These cognitions are typically conceptualised as falling into one of two categories: (1) our conditional beliefs (typically expressed in our attitudes, assumptions, standards and rules for living) and (2) our unconditional beliefs (the core beliefs which reflect a person's fundamental ideas about who they are and how the world operates).

Conditional and unconditional beliefs are closely linked in that a person's attitudes, assumptions, standards and rules usually emerge from their core beliefs. In practice, therapists usually address these levels separately, often targeting conditional beliefs first as these are generally easier to modify.

When should therapists work with enduring cognitions?

We all hold a variety of assumptions, rules for living, standards and core beliefs about how the world works and, although some may be more helpful to us than others, our less adaptive ones may not necessarily result in significant levels of distress or psychopathology. Moreover, it would be neither helpful nor time-efficient to try to target all of these. Enduring cognitions also take longer to modify than automatic thoughts and so an important question for the therapist is when enduring cognitions should become a focus of the therapy and when they should not.

Where a therapist believes that this type of work is likely to prove beneficial, it is usually introduced when a client fully understands the CBT approach, appreciates how their cognitions can be biased and has

Table 6.1. Guidelines for when to work with enduring cognitions

A persistent thought emerges in the way the client tells their story, suggesting that it is arising from a more deeply-held belief.	✓
Therapist and client identify a particular theme in the client's thought records.	✓
The client is good at modifying their NATs but, despite this, the same NAT or variation of it consistently recurs.	✓
The client describes two or three presenting problems that seem linked by a more fundamental belief or concern.	✓
The client makes good progress in working towards their goals and no longer experiences distress. Nonetheless, the therapist and client identify a more deeply-held cognition that, if left unattended, could leave the client vulnerable to difficulties in the future.	✓
When asked to rate on a 0–100% scale how strongly the client believes what the therapist suspects is an enduring cognition, the rating is very high.	✓
The cognition, when expressed, causes the client distress, difficulty or otherwise limits the client's options or is preventing the client from achieving their therapy objectives.	✓
The cognition is unhelpfully absolutist, rigid, unrelenting and dominant rather than representing one idea within a broader range of more adaptive beliefs.	✓

had experience of successfully modifying their automatic thoughts. Other signs that working with enduring cognitions may be helpful are included in Table 6.1.

Orienting clients to working with enduring cognitions

Clients need a rationale for modifying their enduring cognitions so that they can collaborate in the process of working at this level and in using the interventions to which the therapist introduces them. Providing clients with a rationale typically begins with psychoeducation. As described in previous chapters, an important message that underpins CBT is that our beliefs are learned rather than being objective realities. What we learn will be the product of many influences throughout our lives. From the time we are born, we actively try to make sense of our world as we discover how to get our fundamental needs met for love, care and nurturing. The environment in which we grow up will have a profound impact on what we learn about the world. For example, a child who grows up in a family home with caregivers who are able to offer consistent care, love and protection and who can provide enough material resources for the child to be well-fed, warm and safe will likely learn a number of fundamental 'truths', such as:

- I am safe and loved
- Others are trustworthy, reliable and caring
- The world is safe and life is (generally) good

In contrast, a child who grows up in a family where one parent has a mental health problem, where both parents fight regularly under the influence of alcohol and the child is neglected emotionally and physically is likely to arrive at conclusions such as:

- I am unsafe and unloved
- Others are unpredictable and untrustworthy
- The world is dangerous and life is difficult

These enduring cognitions, formed in the context of their life experiences, provide each child with different templates for future relationships and behaviour. The first child will likely acquire a stable base from which to explore their world and to learn and grow. Over time, their beliefs about the world will be elaborated. This child will need to learn that not everyone can be trusted and that life is not always good, but a stable point of departure provides the child with the basis for secure self-esteem. In contrast, the second child will likely grow up with doubts about their own security and worth, a belief that others are unreliable and a view that the world is dangerous. It is not difficult to anticipate the implications for emotional well-being that these different cognitive templates might have.

Helping clients appreciate that their deeply-held beliefs might be something that they have learned creates some interesting possibilities for exploration and change. First, anything that is learned can be examined for its current validity (how accurate it is now), its historical validity (it might have been true once but may not be any more), conceptualised empathically (it is understandable that a client would have arrived at certain beliefs given their personal history and environment); tested (just because something is understandable it doesn't necessarily follow that it is true; the belief needs to be tested to determine its accuracy) and, where appropriate, revised in light of new information (through a process of evidence-gathering using some of the methods outlined in this and the other chapters in this book). These different stages of modifying enduring cognitions are considered next.

Eliciting and modifying conditional beliefs

Conditional beliefs comprise a range of cognitions that we acquire to help us navigate our way through life. These cognitions principally comprise assumptions (i.e. beliefs about what the self, others and the world are actually like), standards (i.e. beliefs about how things *should* be) and rules for living (i.e. how to get by in life given the way the world works).

There are several ways in which therapists can identify a client's conditional beliefs. These include:

1. Listening for examples in how the client describes their experience.
2. Looking for themes that emerge through a process of guided discovery.

3. Observing patterns in a client's thought records that suggest the presence of a more deeply-held belief.
4. Asking the client directly about the assumptions, standards and rules that they hold.
5. Using downward arrowing (see Chapter 5).

Strategies for working with conditional beliefs include the following:

- Helping the client develop an empathic understanding about the origins of an unhelpful conditional belief
- Examining the advantages and disadvantages of living life according to an unhelpful conditional belief
- Developing a new, more adaptive conditional belief
- Using behavioural experiments to test predictions associated with an old and/or new conditional belief (this can sometimes take the form of encouraging the client to act as if the new belief were true in order to observe the consequences)

In the next case study, we consider how some of these methods might be applied to Amber, a client working with CBT therapist Rene for long-standing, recurrent depression and low self-esteem.

Case study: Amber

In working together over time, Rene and Amber noticed that one particular cognition kept appearing in Amber's thought records: namely, the belief (in this case, a standard) that, "If I make a mistake, it means I am worthless", which Amber believed to be 100% true.

Rene helped Amber identify several noteworthy qualities of this standard. First, it seemed rigid and absolute, reflecting an 'all-or-nothing' reasoning bias. Second, this standard seemed to conflate self-worth with performance in a way that was problematic. Third, living life according to this standard seemed to be costing Amber a great deal. In particular, it robbed her of the joy of learning and constrained her opportunities to learn and grow. Not surprisingly, Amber had difficulties with being spontaneous; the idea of trying new things was threatening to her and she was typically highly distressed by setbacks, perceiving them as 'proof' of her worthlessness.

Amber was able to locate the origins of her unhelpful standard in her school years. Her parents, successful academics, had heavily promoted the value of learning and the opportunities to which hard work could give rise. Amber wanted to please her parents and she saw academic attainment as a way of securing their regard. She said she had not been naturally gifted but had managed to secure good grades through implementing a rigid and unforgiving study schedule that excluded 'wasted time' for friendships and hobbies. The praise she received for her academic success from her parents and teachers helped cement her belief that she was valuable only if she excelled, and reinforced her approach to learning. Thus, the positive message her parents had intended to give became problematically intertwined with her self-worth.

In working with this standard over a period of months and drawing on the interventions described above, Rene initially helped Amber consolidate her own understanding of why she had formed this belief using the summary sheet shown in Figure 6.1.

The problematic standard that I want to change is...

"If I make a mistake, it means I am worthless" (I initially believed this 100%)

It is understandable that I have held this standard because...

It relates to lessons that I learned about academic success and self-worth when I was young. I was afraid that I would disappoint my parents if I didn't excel, so I over-worked to make sure that I didn't let them down. I began to see their approval as dependent on my success. Over time, I concluded that I was only of any value if I excelled and so making mistakes felt very threatening.

This standard has been helpful to me because...

1.   At school, I did better than I could have ever imagined.
2.   I learned early in life what hard work could help me accomplish, so I've always been willing to push myself.
3.   I'm good at organising myself and planning my time.
4.   I don't procrastinate in the way that other people seem to struggle with; I can easily motivate myself to do what I need to do.
5.   I have a job that I love because I worked so hard to get it.

However, this standard has been unhelpful to me because....

1.   At school I became a recluse because I was studying all the time.
2.   I was robbed of the joy of learning. Studying became a source of worry rather than a source of pleasure and satisfaction.
3.   It makes me anxious and unhappy. I suspect that this belief has a role to play in my depression and low self-esteem.
4.   I am so afraid of making mistakes that I avoid trying new things.
5.   I am highly sensitive to criticism. I can't accept feedback, even when I know that it is well intentioned, because I see it as a sign that I have failed.

Figure 6.1.   Amber's re-evaluation of her original standard

Having drawn together all this information into a summary, Amber could better understand why she had developed this standard for herself while at the same time appreciating that it had cost her a great deal. She was then willing to work with Rene to identify a new and more helpful standard.

If it was to prove persuasive to Amber, Rene understood that any new standard would need to accommodate the perceived benefits of the old one while also offering greater flexibility.

Following discussion, a new potential standard, worthy of testing, was identified as follows: *"If I want to fulfil my potential, then I need to learn and grow and sometimes this will mean making mistakes."*

Amber initially rated her belief in this statement at only 50%, but she recognised how this new standard could potentially introduce greater flexibility into her life. So, with the help of Rene, she constructed the following series of experiments to test out the validity and helpfulness of this new standard.

Desk-based research

Amber identified ten individuals throughout history whom she regarded as having been undeniably successful. She researched the biographies of these individuals to learn more about their histories and accomplishments. She was surprised to discover that all of them had encountered substantial difficulties in their lives and careers. Some had experienced bankruptcy, others had had to fight legal battles, some had been cast out by the societies in which they lived, and others had had to persist in the face of repeated failures.

Amber's conclusion: If I go by the experience of those I admire, making mistakes and struggling does not mean failure. In fact, the more successful people have been, the more struggles they are likely to have experienced along the way.

New belief rating: 60%

Strategic risk-taking

Amber then decided to test out putting herself in situations that she would usually avoid for fear of making a mistake. Two of these experiments were as follows:

Amber volunteered for a work-related project on an area of her company's business with which she was less familiar. In the weeks that followed, she kept a log of (1) her perceived sense of contribution to the project, (2) feedback on her contribution, and (3) her levels of discomfort. She discovered that, despite her predictions, she enjoyed the project and was able to make an important contribution. Her suggestions were not always accepted by the group and on two occasions she felt she had asked "stupid questions". Nonetheless, both she and her line manager received positive feedback about her contribution from the project manager.

Amber's conclusion: Although I felt nervous and out of my depth to begin with, the anxiety eased over time. I learned that I had something valuable to contribute and this was appreciated even though my lack of knowledge in some areas meant that I sometimes got things wrong. I enjoyed being part of this project and gave myself the chance to learn and grow.

New belief rating: 80%

At her appraisal, she decided to ask how her line manager perceived Amber's future within the company. Her manager was candid in her response, saying that while she saw potential for promotion, Amber had not sufficiently engaged with opportunities for building her knowledge, skills and profile. She also said that she had found Amber defensive when given constructive feedback. Her manager said that she would be happy to work with Amber to formulate a plan that would help her work towards promotion but that this would not be forthcoming until Amber had addressed these areas.

This feedback was difficult for Amber to hear, initially evoking the sense of failure that she so greatly feared. Yet she could now appreciate that this was precisely the type of feedback that would enable her to learn and grow. She recognised that her manager saw her potential and had simply stated what needed to occur for Amber to be promoted. This enabled her to begin to develop an action plan with which her line manager was pleased to support her.

Amber's conclusion: If I am to fulfil my potential, I need to be open to feedback (even when it is uncomfortable to hear). My manager clearly wants to help me develop my career and I can use her feedback to become more open to new experiences that will help me progress in the way that I want.

New belief rating: 85%

These, and other interventions of this kind, took place over an extended period as Amber accumulated and reflected upon the information gathered at each stage. Gradually, she learned to modify her understanding of success and failure. She concluded that mistakes were a sign she was learning and growing, that just because something is uncomfortable does not mean it is bad, and that her value as a human being did not depend on how she performed on any individual task. At the end of therapy, she believed her new standard 100% and was committed to applying it to every aspect of her life.

Eliciting and modifying unconditional beliefs

Embedded within assumptions, standards and rules for living are our core beliefs – those most deeply-held cognitions about who we are as individuals, how relationships work and the ways of the world at large. Like conditional beliefs, core beliefs are not always readily expressed by clients. This may be because they are not immediately obvious to the client or are assumed to simply reflect the way the world is and so are not worthy of reflection. The therapist, then, needs to remain alert to the presence of core beliefs in how a client tells their story and is likely to build up a picture of these over time rather than during a first meeting.

Although they can take many forms, J. S. Beck (2011) suggests that the problematic, absolutist core beliefs with which CBT therapists are concerned tend to fall into one or two broad categories (sometimes both): (1) those relating to helplessness and (2) those relating to unlovability. She highlights that it is not always obvious to the therapist which category of belief a client is describing. For example, if a client refers to a sense of themselves as defective, this may refer to a belief about helplessness (e.g. not being as good, strong, resourceful, competent or effective as others) or unlovability (e.g. being different, odd, abnormal or damaged and unlovable as a result). This is one of the reasons why developing an understanding of the client's core beliefs takes time and why ensuring that the therapist's choice of strategies is underpinned by a formulation, which we describe in Chapter 10, is critical.

The methods used for identifying core beliefs are similar to those used for uncovering assumptions, standards and rules for living. For example, core beliefs can be identified through the use of guided discovery and downward arrowing and patterns in a client's thought records (see Chapter 5) and asking the client directly about the beliefs that they hold in relation to themselves, others, relationships and the world around them. Sometimes asking a client to list their responses to the statements "I am ...", "Other people/relationships are ..." and "The world/life is ..." can yield useful information for subsequent exploration.

The seed of a relevant core belief can also be implicit in a person's conditional beliefs. For example, in the case of Amber, described above, her original unhelpful standard, "If I make a mistake, it means I am worthless", could indicate the presence of a core belief, "I am worthless", which her therapist might then choose to explore.

When helping the client develop a new core belief, it is important to include not only those qualities that are more adaptive but also those that permit greater flexibility with room for the client to be 'only human'. For example, a therapist would not encourage a client who once held the belief, "I am a failure" to construct the new belief "I am perfect", as this new belief is just as extreme, absolutist and rigid as the old one. The qualities of any new belief can, then, include words such as 'generally', 'most of the time', 'I'm/it's OK'. Thus, the core belief, "I am a failure", might become "I am successful on many levels" and the belief, "I am bad", might become "I am generally a good person but I'm only human".

When therapist and client have arrived at a belief that seems desirable for the client, the therapist will need to choose a strategy that can help the client gather evidence to support their new, more realistic belief and weaken the influence of the former, unhelpful one. In the example at the start of this chapter we described the core beliefs of a client who had grown up in a family where one parent had a mental health problem, both parents were fighting under the influence of alcohol and the child was neglected emotionally and physically. Helping the client appreciate that a child growing up in such an environment would have almost inevitably concluded that they were unsafe and unloved, that others are unpredictable and untrustworthy, and that the world is dangerous can support the client in restructuring these early beliefs. This may include recording memories that contributed to the core belief, searching for evidence that supports the new, positive belief for each period of the client's life and reframing each piece of evidence for the old belief to take account of what the client now knows.

Points to remember about enduring cognitions

Although it is always important for the client to understand the rationale for the methods that the therapist is using, this is particularly important when working with enduring cognitions. Not all enduring cognitions are hard to shift but, generally, our beliefs tend to be more resistant to change than our automatic thoughts. As a result, any strategies applied usually need to be used over a period of months before the client notices consistent improvement. It is vital, therefore, that the client understands what the process of modifying problematic beliefs will entail so that they do not lose heart when change is not instant.

Conclusion

This chapter has sought to further illustrate the complexity of our cognitive world by introducing when, why and how a CBT therapist might work with enduring cognitions. The aim has been to introduce some of the most commonly used interventions and illustrate how they build upon the methods typically used earlier in therapy, which we have described in other chapters. Although working at this level may not always be necessary, our enduring cognitions are a powerful mediator of how we feel, think and behave. Where the client's needs suggest that this is indicated, the strategies introduced in this chapter provide a sound, theoretically- and clinically-informed basis for intervention.

Reflective Activity: Working with one of your standards

Select a standard that you hold that you think is worthy of reflection. This might be because you sense that it carries some costs as well as benefits or because it is a standard that has shaped your life in a powerful way. Then consider your responses using the following prompts:

- The standard that I am interested in examining and that may benefit from some refinement is ...
- It is understandable that I have held this belief because ...
- This belief has been helpful to me because ...
- However, this belief has, or may have, been unhelpful to me because ...
- If I were going to modify this standard in a way that retained its benefits but introduced greater flexibility or new possibilities, what would this be?
- If I wanted to try out this new, adapted standard what might I do? What actions might I take and what experiments might I conduct to see what impact this revised standard might have on my life?

Interested in learning more? Check out ...

Simmons, J., & Griffiths, R. (2014). *CBT for beginners* (2nd ed.). London: SAGE.

SEVEN

Working with Imagery

Chapter objectives

By reading this chapter you will be able to:

- Understand why working with imagery is important in CBT
- Know how a CBT therapist might approach eliciting a client's images
- Describe some of the strategies used to modify unhelpful images and develop adaptive ones

Introduction

In the earlier chapters that considered the cognitive strategies which CBT therapists typically use, the focus was on working with cognitions as verbal statements: that is, automatic thoughts, conditional beliefs and unconditional beliefs. However, we do not always think in verbal statements. There is another category of cognition that is powerful both in terms of maintaining clients' distress and in providing a pathway to change: namely, imagery.

Imagery has been implicated in a variety of common mental health problems and emotional difficulties, as well as in their treatment and recovery. Not surprisingly, then, CBT therapists are increasingly called upon to work with clients' imagery and need to have the skills and strategies to do so effectively.

This chapter examines how CBT understands the role of imagery in emotional distress and its resolution. We begin by examining the nature of imagery and why working with clients' images can be so important. We then look at some of the ways in which therapists go about eliciting their clients' images before introducing some of the most commonly used strategies to enable emotional well-being and behaviour change.

What is imagery?

As human beings we make sense of life through the images we create as well as through our thoughts, assumptions, standards and beliefs. Our imagery includes a variety of internal, visually-based experiences that take the form of mental pictures, fantasy scenarios and 'mental movies'. They can have a basis in reality, as is the case when we go back into memory, or be entirely fictitious, as in the case of fantasy.

Images can be fleeting and at times difficult to identify. While some clients readily identify themselves as 'visual thinkers' others find it difficult to recognise the mental pictures that might be present and bound up with episodes of difficulty or distress. Other images can be intrusive, difficult to control or feel embarrassing or shameful to share. This was illustrated in the case of Sandy in Chapter 2, who was struggling with intrusive images of hurting others in the context of obsessive-compulsive disorder. In such cases, without an understanding of what their presence does and does not mean, these images are likely to give rise to feelings of anxiety and to negative automatic thoughts, such as: "I can't control my mind"; "I am an evil person"; "If I tell my therapist she might report me to the police".

Images, then, can occur spontaneously, arising unbidden in our minds without any effort or desire on our part (intrusive images), while others can be consciously courted (picturing oneself on an idyllic desert island having just won the lottery). Some can be enjoyable to indulge and make us feel good, whereas others can be highly distressing and difficult to share due to a fear of how we might be judged.

Why work with images?

Images matter because they are bound up with our automatic thoughts, our emotional and physical responses and how we act and react in any given situation. Working with images can bridge the so-called head–heart lag that clients can sometimes experience when modifying their negative automatic thoughts (see Chapter 5). For many people, images feel more connected to their emotions than do verbal cognitions, and there is some evidence that images impact the body, our thinking and our behaviour in unique ways. Consider, for example, the disorders and images listed in Table 7.1. How would you predict that these images would make a person feel emotionally and physically and to what types of thoughts and behaviours might they give rise?

Table 7.1.   Images associated with common mental health problems

Panic attacks:	An image of oneself having collapsed on the floor, unable to breathe and clutching one's chest in agony
Social anxiety:	An image of oneself at a party with others pointing at one, frowning and then laughing
Body dysmorphia:	An image of oneself as ugly, deformed and grotesque
OCD:	An image of oneself stabbing a loved one in the absence of any desire or intention to do so
Health anxiety:	An image of one's children at one's funeral
Spider phobia:	An image of an enormous spider charging across the floor towards the person with a mean look on its face
Phobia of flying:	An image of the plane diving through the sky about to crash, with all the passengers crying and screaming

In reading through the list in Table 7.1, you may have identified that these distressing images contain elements that are not entirely accurate. For example, in our experience, spiders rarely have 'mean looks on their faces'! You might also have identified other ways in which each of the images described is, or could potentially be, subtly distorted as problematic images tend to contain the same reasoning biases that are contained in negative automatic thoughts (see Chapter 2). Understanding that our images do not represent an objective account of a situation provides therapists with a clue as to what to look for when a client is distressed and the kinds of modifications that may be required.

How to elicit images

Where a therapist suspects that images are an important part of the clinical picture, a first step involves knowing how to identify them. One approach to uncovering images is simply to ask about their presence as a client tells their story – particularly when strong emotions are present. As discussed in Chapter 2, therapists often attempt to better understand a client's cognitive world by asking, "At that moment when you felt so bad, what went through your mind?" This question is equally valid for uncovering images.

It is also useful to think about having a broad vocabulary when talking with clients about imagery-based experiences. As J. S. Beck (2011) reminds us, the term 'imagery' may not resonate with a client so it is important to have a range of alternatives which a client might better understand. She suggests that therapists familiarise themselves with synonyms, such as mental pictures, daydreams, imagining and memories. In our experience, using phrases like, "Can you paint the scene for me?" and, "Help me get a picture in my mind of what you experienced", and asking clients about any mental movies they were seeing in their mind's eye can also be useful prompts.

Where the therapist senses that a client is experiencing images that are uncomfortable to disclose, a further way of making them safe to share is psychoeducation. For example, unpleasant, intrusive images are a frequent experience for people living with OCD and post-traumatic stress disorder. However, clients will probably not be aware that a very high proportion of the general population also experiences intrusive thoughts. Our minds, it seems, are naturally inclined towards serving up images that are at times unsettling, frightening, violent or just bizarre, and helping clients understand this can go a long way to reducing feelings of embarrassment and shame.

An analogy that can be helpful is likening images to an email inbox. Similar to emails, some images are important and need our attention. Others are entertaining but potentially distracting so we need to attend to them when we have the time to indulge them. Other images are like email spam: neither important nor useful. Spam emails can take different forms but when we see them, we do not worry about them, fear them or feel judged because they are there. We simply recognise them for what they are and delete them. We can apply the same approach to our images. Using this analogy alongside psychoeducation can help a client appreciate that images are a normal part of cognition and that the therapist is unlikely to be shocked by what the client is visualising.

Some clients may be willing to share their images but need help in recognising when imagery-based experiences are occurring. This is often a matter of practice. One way of helping a client connect with their images is to ask them to describe a recent neutral scene or situation (e.g. travelling to see the therapist) or familiar object (e.g. their living room). These tasks – which most people can do relatively easy – cannot be accomplished without conjuring up a mental picture, so if a client is able to do this, they are able to access their images.

In order to access images that are implicated in a client's difficulties, a therapist might encourage a client to "talk me through the distressing situation, picturing it clearly in your mind and describing the details". Where aspects of the image seem to be absent or require elaboration, the therapist can direct the client to providing more information about colours, sound (in the case of a mental movie), light, size and the shape of different aspects.

Once a client has a sense of the images that are relevant for them and has practised this in the session with their therapist, they are likely to be asked to do some imagery-based homework. The therapist might ask the client to track when problematic images are occurring and to make a note of where and when they occur using an adapted version of the thought record introduced in Chapter 5. Alternatively, the therapist might encourage identifying images that are present when the client experiences automatic thoughts to help elicit connections between the client's verbal and visual cognitions.

As for thoughts and behaviours, merely tracking images can start to introduce changes. Yet for most clients this is only the first step. The next step involves modifying distressing images and creating more positive ones.

Strategies for changing images

The images we experience are mental constructions. Even where they are based on a memory of something that actually occurred, images live inside our heads. In this sense, they are 'made up'. This is good news because it means that images can be changed and that we can experiment with changes without any risk to ourselves or others.

Consider how we can alter our images and how we might experience them differently as a result (all the following might be used within CBT and you might like to experiment with them yourself). For example, we can:

- Shrink or enlarge an image
- Change the colour of an image or drain it of colour (a sepia image may not feel quite as distressing or convincing as one in rich and vivid colours)
- Place ourselves inside an image (i.e. make ourselves part of the scene)
- Stand outside the image (i.e. adopt the perspective of an observer)
- Add or remove an item within the image that changes its emotional impact (e.g. introduce an enormous cuddly teddy bear into a frightening image)
- Alter the size of characters or objects within the image (e.g. shrink an aggressive person to a miniature size with a squeaky voice)
- Make an image stationary, like a photograph

- Create a mental movie to which we can add or remove a soundtrack, and which we can play in slow motion or at double speed
- Run a distressing mental movie backwards
- Create an image of a safe place to which we can return in our minds whenever we feel anxious or afraid

All the above have potential implications for how we relate to the image and its emotional and physical impact. Used in therapy, the therapist would be interested in exploring what the client experienced as a result of the changes they made, as illustrated in the case study below.

Case study: Keira

Keira's long-standing low self-esteem and sense of powerlessness in her life had been reinforced by a former boss who had continually shouted at and undermined her. Although Keira had long since left this job, the memory of what had occurred – played out inside her head as a mental movie – continued to haunt her. Keira's therapist, Maryam, was interested in finding out if Keira felt any different because of modifying this mental movie.

Maryam: What was that like for you, Keira – going back to that painful image of your old boss putting you down in the way he used to but this time introducing some changes?

Keira: Interesting ... It felt different somehow ...

Maryam: Different ... how? Can you put into words what that felt like for you?

Keira: I guess it had never occurred to me that I could change the image. I thought I was stuck with it. After all, those things did happen.

Maryam: That's important, isn't it? Even if it is based on something that happened in real life, an image is something that we create in our minds. If we don't like what we are creating, we can create something different.

Keira: Hmm. In the past, I tried to deal with the image by pushing it out of my mind but that never really worked. But this felt ... somehow I felt stronger.

Maryam: So let's recap on what we did there. You began by describing what the image was like: a movie that you were running inside your head that was in full colour, with your old boss a huge figure in the film, screaming at you. What did you do then?

Keira: You asked me to turn down the volume on my boss's voice until the image became silent. And then you said to drain the colour so that it looked like an old, black-and-white silent movie.

Maryam: What difference, if any, did that make?

Keira: It made the movie feel very old – like it happened a long time in the past which made it feel less personal and less frightening.

Maryam: Then what did you do?
Keira: You suggested that I add a soundtrack, like one of those tinkling piano scores used to accompany the old silent movies.
Maryam: Anything else?
Keira: (slight giggle) I turned my old boss into one of those villains that you used to see in the silent movies. I put a pantomime moustache on him, added some heavy make-up like the actors used to wear and had him cavorting around the set.
Maryam: So you really did turn this into an old silent movie! (laughs)
Keira: (laughs also) I guess I did! I've always enjoyed those old films – Charlie Chaplin, Buster Keaton, Harold Lloyd – they always make me laugh.
Maryam: Sounds like you hit on something that really resonated with you. And what impact did that have – turning the frightening image into one of those old movies that you really enjoy?
Keira: I stopped being afraid. It was comical somehow. Just for that moment, I stopped being afraid of the past.
Maryam: So how about you practise this between now and when we next meet. Whenever that frightening and disempowering image comes to mind, prac-tise transforming it into an old black-and-white movie, silencing the shout-ing, draining the colour and adding a piano soundtrack and not, of course, forgetting the villain's stage make-up! (Keira and Maryam both laugh)

Here, Maryam is teaching Keira that she can purposefully manipulate a distressing image in ways that are more adaptive to Keira's circumstances and needs. Although this is not the only intervention that Maryam will use, and therapy will need to help Keira address a number of areas of her life, Keira is learning that she can modify her images even when they are based on real-life events. This can be an important basis for enabling a sense of empowerment in the context of a painful past.

As with all CBT interventions, the choice of approach will depend on what the therapist is wanting to achieve. Is it to educate the client about the power of imagery? To modify distressing images that occur spontane-ously or to help the client create new images for the purposes of cognitive restructuring? Is it to help them rehearse a more adaptive response to a previously anxiety-provoking situation or to use imagery rehearsal for an important event, such as a work interview or preparing for a forthcoming flight in the case of a fear of flying?

Depending on the rationale for its use, there are two broad categories of intervention with which the therapist is concerned. The first category involves addressing distressing or problematic images – those that typically arise spontaneously in the client's mind. The second is where the therapist teaches the client how to induce positive imagery to support the pursuit of desired objectives. In the next section we introduce some of the strategies used for each of these categories in turn.

Transforming problematic images

In modifying distressing, spontaneously occurring images, J. S. Beck (2011) has identified three primary interventions: (1) following images to completion, (2) moving forward in time, and (3) introducing coping into the image. The first and second of these interventions address the tendency that clients have to halt their images at the worst possible moment. For example, the person experiencing panic attacks ends the image at the point where they see themselves being unable to breathe or having a heart attack – not in the safety of a hospital bed being reassured by a doctor that this was a panic attack and that the tests reveal that the client has a healthy heart. Equally, if a client has been given a poor grade for their appraisal, they are more likely to visualise losing their job than imagining their boss providing a subsequent positive appraisal based on the client taking on board the previous year's feedback.

J. S. Beck (2011) suggests that when people follow through their images to completion the person will either visualise themselves getting through the crisis, with the associated reduction in distress, or anticipate a further catastrophe. Where the latter occurs, it is an opportunity to explore what happens next, which is likely to be another visualised catastrophe that can also be modified, either through following the image through to completion or through moving the image into the future.

A client might be helped to modify a problematic image by moving forward in time to a point at which the situation has resolved. Unlike the strategy of following an image through to completion, this may involve the client looking ahead to a point over the longer term, at which the situation has resolved itself. For example, university student Ed was struggling with a catastrophic image of freezing in his first-year exams. Whenever he sat at his desk, this image would present itself and was interfering with his ability to revise. His therapist suggested that Ed run the image forward in time to the point at which he graduated, imagining himself celebrating with his friends and recollecting how tough his first year of revision had been but how glad he was that he had persisted with his studies.

Sometimes a problematic image is most usefully modified by the therapist introducing imaginal coping. This involves taking the client through the image, step by step, and as something difficult occurs, encouraging them to consider what they might do to manage the situation. That method of coping is then introduced into the image and might include the strategies that a client has learned in therapy, such as controlled breathing, modifying negative automatic thoughts or using social skills as described in Chapter 7. This can help the client discover that the situation is manageable and draw their attention to strategies they have already used, that they might imagine themselves using and other coping or rescue factors that reduce the distressing or catastrophic nature of a problematic image.

A final intervention that can be useful is altering the perspective from which the client experiences the image. As noted previously, we can place ourselves inside an image or outside the image looking in. Here, a therapist might ask a client to imagine the scene unfolding as though it were taking place on the set of a movie. The client is asked to position themselves behind the director and to notice the camera operators, sound engineers and stagehands in attendance. At the conclusion of the scene, the director says "cut" and then everyone claps in agreement that the scene was well acted. A variation of this method can be the client imagining themselves projecting a distressing mental picture on to a television screen. They then imagine themselves watching the scene and then reaching for the remote control and turning off the television, perhaps even turning to a family member sitting beside them in the image and remarking that it was "a bad film and a waste of our time watching it".

Inducing positive imagery

In addition to modifying unhelpful imagery, the therapist might also use positive imagery to enable desired states. In such circumstances, in contrast to working with distressing images that are spontaneously arising, the therapist will encourage the client to design and then practise conjuring up images that are positively impactful.

There are several forms that positive imagery might take. In the previous section we considered how introducing coping into the image can be a way of helping the client rehearse challenging situations using methods of problem-solving that can create a sense of empowerment. In the field of compassionate mind therapy, Lee (2005) writes about the use of imagery to help clients conjure up a 'perfect nurturer' – a fantasy figure whose qualities provide everything that the client needs in terms of acceptance, caring, wisdom, strength and support. Padesky (1994) has described how role-play can be used to reconstruct the meaning of historically problematic interpersonal interactions.

An additional intervention is one recommended by Padeksy (2005) where a client creates an image of how they would like things to be. This can be a powerful approach to helping clients construct mental images that support a process of moving towards a desired outcome. Clients are encouraged to make these images as compelling as possible. As we discussed earlier in this chapter, the impact of our images is affected by their qualities – a photograph or a movie, black and white or colour, being inside or outside the image. In designing a desirable image, the therapist will help the client to identify qualities that help make the image feel as vivid and convincing as possible. The therapist will then encourage the client to explore, in detail, their behaviours in this desired image and ask them to consider the types of automatic thoughts, conditional and unconditional beliefs that they might need to make this desired future possible.

The mental rehearsal of desired states can be powerful. Athletes and performing artists sometimes use this strategy to help prepare psychologically for important competitive events or other kinds of performances. This type of covert rehearsal can also be helpful when we are building up to a desired but anxiety-provoking event, such as a presentation, job interview or other challenging, growth-promoting experience.

Points to remember

Images can be tested for their accuracy through use of the evidence-gathering methods described elsewhere in this book. Nonetheless, where a client is experiencing mental pictures, imagery-based interventions are generally more effective than verbal techniques such as thought records.

Like the other strategies described in this book, imagery-based techniques tend to require ongoing practice. They may also involve a degree of trial and error to discover which methods are optimally helpful for a client's needs. As Kennerley et al. (2017) also remind us, the mental pictures we create are often powerful. Encouraging clients to engage with their imagery can therefore evoke strong emotional and physical reactions. One example of this is where a client has experienced trauma or abuse. It is important, therefore, always to work at the client's pace and to consider the client's overall resilience and repertoire of coping skills before proceeding. This can help the therapist decide on the timing and sequencing of imagery interventions relative to the use of other methods.

Finally, images can also take the form of a 'felt sense' (Gendlin, 1996). At times, a client's experience may not take the form of a specific image but rather an instinctual, bodily reaction to a specific situation or event. The therapist will therefore want to be alert to the different ways in which a client's experience might manifest itself. Where a more visceral reaction occurs, it is important to help the client find ways to put their experience into words in order to identify potential avenues for intervention.

Conclusion

The adage that 'a picture is worth a thousand words' sums up the experience of many clients whose difficulties appear to be fuelled more by mental images than by thoughts, assumptions or beliefs. Yet, like verbal cognitions, problematic images often contain the cognitive biases we examined in Chapter 2, can be subjected to reality testing and, where appropriate, modified in ways that are helpful.

Because they take place inside our heads, images are by definition mental phenomena rather than objective realities. This means that the client, guided by the therapist, can be encouraged to experiment with their imagery to see what results this might produce. Our minds are endlessly creative and, regardless of which strategy the therapist uses, there is the potential to use imagery to identify new and more helpful possibilities for the client's future and to experiment with these before taking them into the real world.

As the field has evolved, CBT has expanded its range of imagery-based strategies to address specific clinical problems. Examples would include interventions such as reliving and imagery rescripting for working with PTSD, traumatic grief and early abuse. While these are important innovations, they take us beyond the introductory scope of this book, where the focus is on those strategies that form the therapist's general toolbox. Nonetheless, whether the purpose is to access unhelpful cognitions, modify distressing images or install more helpful images that support a client in working towards a desired future, the variety of ways in which we can manipulate the pictures inside our heads gives us a rich array of options for experimenting with new ways of thinking and acting.

Reflective Activity: Using imagery to help achieve your goal

Think of a goal that you have for yourself. It could be in relation to any area of your life. Create an image of yourself having achieved your goal. Make the image as compelling, detailed and life-like as possible using the ideas introduced in this chapter. What thoughts, assumptions, beliefs and behaviours would need to be present to help you achieve your goal? Can you identify any steps that you might now want to take to move closer to this desired outcome?

Interested in Learning More? Check out ...

Beck, J. S. (2020). *Cognitive behavior therapy: Basics and beyond* (3rd ed.). New York: Guilford Press.

EIGHT

Behavioural Methods for Building Skills and Changing Patterns of Activity

Chapter objectives

By reading this chapter you will be able to:

- Name and describe some of the main behavioural interventions that are used in CBT
- Understand the difference between skills-based methods and guided behaviour change
- Explain when and why skills training is likely to be used in CBT
- Explain when and why behavioural activation is important to use in CBT

Introduction

It is one thing to create change at the cognitive level, but quite another thing to implement actual changes in how we live. This chapter considers the implications of the behavioural principle introduced in Chapter 3 for the use of specific methods and how these might be introduced to a client and implemented within therapy.

There is an extensive range of behavioural methods upon which CBT therapists can draw in the service of helping a client achieve meaningful change. As a comprehensive overview is beyond the scope of this book, we have chosen in this chapter to focus on two broad categories of behavioural intervention that feature prominently in many forms of CBT application. These are: (1) skills-based methods, that is, interventions that involve a skills component that the client needs to learn and practise in pursuit of a desired objective or life direction, and (2) guided behaviour change, that is, where the client is directed towards changing aspects of their behaviour in order to create a more favourable outcome. Examples of each of these are considered in turn.

Skills training

One of the challenges to the psychotherapy movement in general, and to which behavioural approaches have sought to provide a solution, is the importance of ensuring that clients acquire the life skills they need to enable them to live effectively in the world. The recognition that talking therapies do not necessarily lead to changes in how clients are able to function has led to skills training becoming a major focus for CBT therapists.

In general, behavioural methods for building skills are concerned with assisting individuals in becoming more skilful in identified areas of their lives as well as changing the activity within the system of which they are a part. In this chapter we focus on two among several possible areas of skills training that CBT therapists frequently use: (1) social skills training, which covers a broad range of interventions; and (2) skills in emotion regulation.

Training in social skills

Social skills deficits are an important part of many emotional and behavioural difficulties for children, adolescents and adults, impacting negatively on their mental health (Spence, 2003). Behavioural methods of value include the direct teaching of specific skills, the modelling of appropriate behaviours, the reinforcement of skills performed and the rehearsal of desired behaviours with feedback.

Social skills training typically progresses through the following stages:

Preliminary steps

- The therapist develops, in conjunction with those who will be taking part in the social skills training, a list of the main problem situations, critical incidents or concerns, which are explored in detail.
- The most effective skills for dealing with the primary issues are identified. It is important to note that social skills training does not comprise a generic package of techniques but represents a carefully structured framework where specific interventions are selected to meet the defined need.
- The skill to be acquired is broken down into a series of smaller steps, each of which can be taught, practised and refined.

Once these preliminary stages are complete, the therapist and client can commence with the skills training itself.

Social skills training

- The therapist provides guidance on the skill to be acquired with live demonstrations provided wherever possible. This may be achieved through the therapist demonstrating the skill or through video examples providing positive and negative illustrations of its use.
- The social skill is then practised. If the training is delivered in a group context, there are ample opportunities to practise the skills with others. Practice can also take the form of one-on-one practice with a therapist or the use of training scripts.
- The therapist provides feedback on what was observed. In a group situation, clients can provide feedback to each other. If the session is video-recorded, this can also be reviewed.
- The fourth phase entails practising the skill in real-life situations. In between sessions the client practises the newly acquired skill and then provides feedback to the therapist or group as to the impact. Sometimes it is possible to incorporate feedback from others. For example, a life partner might be asked to provide structured feedback, as might a teacher or care worker. Where a social skills group is used, it might be possible for members to enter selected social situations together and report back on how they each managed.
- Finally, where possible, a follow-up session is arranged to review progress over the longer term and provide a booster session to enhance the skills developed.

This step-by-step framework is typical of social skills training across a range of difficulties. Where the issues that the client faces require enhanced skilful practice, the approach adds much value. However, although this can be a powerful intervention, there are times when change requires more than skills training as there might be behaviours that have to be managed, such as those that inhibit the performance of the skills or compete with them (Spence, 2003). Consequently, social skills training is now often seen as part of a broader repertoire of approaches for working with emotional and behavioural difficulties as well as developmental disorders. It is also combined with skills training in other areas, including emotion regulation.

Training in emotion regulation

A second, frequently used category of skills training is emotion regulation. Emotions act as signals, alerting us to rewards or threats in the environment, but psychological well-being also requires emotional stability. The ability to increase or decrease emotional intensity is critical if we are to respond effectively to the circumstances in which we find ourselves.

Emotion regulation refers to the process by which we influence what we feel and how we experience and act on our feelings. When conducted effectively, it is a means through which we learn to influence the occurrence, intensity, experience and impact of our emotions.

In the context of therapy, some clients are generally effective at regulating their emotions but struggle to do so in a particular situation. For example, if a client has a meeting with someone whom they have long admired but is feeling very anxious and is concerned that they might make a fool of themselves, they may be motivated to cancel the meeting. The therapist might, therefore, seek to teach this client skills to regulate the anxiety in order to attend the event. Other clients experience excessive or unconstrained emotions that are damaging to themselves and others. For some this can represent a disorder in its own right and is often associated with other mental health conditions.

Useful summaries of emotion regulation techniques are widely available. Working from within the framework of dialectical behaviour therapy, McKay et al. (2007), for example, provide guidelines for adults on how to recognise, label and differentiate emotions and how to improve distress tolerance skills. They emphasise skills that include reducing physical vulnerability (e.g. through capitalising on healthy behaviours such as exercise, sleep, managing physical tension through controlled breathing and moderating the use of alcohol), reducing cognitive vulnerability (e.g. learning how to 'unhook' from painful thoughts, using coping statements) and increasing positive emotions (aided through increasing pleasurable behaviours).

For children, strategies include developing a language for identifying and labelling emotions alongside the modelling of appropriate behaviours by key adults and finding effective solutions to personally challenging situations. A further strategy is encouraging the child to delay their response time by refraining from an immediate reaction. For example, in working with groups of children who tended to react instantly to perceived slights or a sense that something was going to be difficult, Lane (1975) developed a technique called Stop and Think. In this method, the children practised using their emotion as a signal that they had to stop and 'do nothing' for 60 seconds. During that time, they thought about the situation and selected an alternative, more adaptive way to respond. The Stop and Think method, alongside variants of such techniques, is still widely used (see McKay et al., 2011).

Emotion regulation skills have been used in a wide range of contexts, such as work with adolescents and their parents, with addictive behaviours, as well as with adults. Of course, at times, we can all respond to emotional signals in less than optimal ways, perhaps avoiding situations when we need to confront them or approaching them when it would be best to step away. Therefore, any work on emotion regulation always needs to be incorporated within a broader treatment plan where skills training is combined with other methods described in this book to enable the delivery of an effective intervention.

In summary, there are a variety of life skills which CBT can help clients acquire. Although the focus here has been on training in social skills and emotion regulation, the processes outlined above can and have been adapted to multiple areas with which people need assistance, including self-care, time management, decision-making and problem-solving. At times, however, the source of a difficulty does not lie in a skills deficit but in how patterns of action (or inaction) shape our world. This is considered next.

Guided behaviour change

In contrast to skills training, guided behaviour change is not concerned with teaching the client new skills but rather with helping them redesign patterns of activity that move them in a valued life direction. In this category of intervention, the therapist does not provide instruction as they might when teaching a skill, but rather shares principles that are relevant to the focus of therapy and works with the client to identify how they might apply them. Examples of guided behaviour change might include looking at ways of redesigning one's week to allow more time for leisure pursuits, redesigning a night-time routine to enhance the likelihood of a good night's sleep and building opportunities for connection and intimacy in a relationship. One intervention within this category that is commonly used in the treatment of depression is behavioural activation.

Behavioural activation

Behavioural activation helps clients become more active and engaged with life by introducing activities that have the potential to improve their mood.

These activities are likely to include those that are pleasurable, those that enable a sense of achievement (often termed 'mastery' tasks) and those that connect clients to what matters most to them (i.e. their core values). They will also include activities that the client may have been avoiding. Any scheduled activities are monitored to examine their effect on the client's mood, the extent to which they have helped the client achieve their goals, and to note any activities still avoided.

Behavioural activation has a long tradition within CBT, although cognitively- and behaviourally-oriented therapies use it for different ends. For example, while the approach is used within behavioural approaches to shape patterns of reinforcement and redesign aspects of a client's daily life, cognitive therapists also use the approach to support cognitive change.

In recent years there has been a growth of interest in behavioural activation as a standalone treatment for depression (see Martell et al., 2013), which is also recommended by the National Institute for Health and Care Excellence (NICE, 2009). In depression, it is common for individuals to experience a loss of energy and motivation, such that they start to withdraw from the world. For some, life can become so difficult that they struggle to get out of bed in the morning. Yet these withdrawal behaviours are problematic. For example, lying in bed results in diminished access to opportunities for success and is likely to result in rumination, confirming a depressed client's worst fears about themselves ("I can't do anything – it's all hopeless"). A therapist might, therefore, develop a hypothesis that the client's current difficulties are being maintained by their patterns of withdrawal, and a second hypothesis that increasing activity might lead to symptomatic improvement. In the next case study, the transcript illustrates how CBT therapist, Amara, might go about introducing this idea to a client and what implications this could have for therapeutic change.

Case study: Dev

Amara: What you are saying makes a lot of sense to me. Things are so difficult at the moment, you feel like you are swimming through treacle most of the time. So of course you are going to feel drawn to staying in bed. Right now, it's the only place where you feel safe and sometimes when you doze off things feel a bit more peaceful. Is that how it happens?

Dev: Yeah ...

Amara: But you were also telling me something else just then. You said that when you lie in bed, your mind churns things over and you end up dwelling on how you believe you have ruined your life. Could you tell me more about that?

Dev: Well, I can't believe it's come to this – that I can't even get out of bed. I used to go to work, accomplish things ... I was a good husband and father. Now look at me.

Amara: (gently) What sort of things go through your mind when you lie in bed dwelling?

Dev: That I'm a failure ... that I've ruined my life. Nothing I do makes any difference. It's all pointless.

Amara: That sounds so painful ...

Dev: (very quietly) I keep waiting to feel better but now I'm starting to worry that I never will ...

Amara: (pauses) I can see why it might seem that way to you ... And yet, you have also told me that there are some days when, somehow, you manage to get yourself out of bed. And you mentioned that when you do, you sometimes feel a little better. I wonder, what's different on those days ...

Dev: It's not always the case, but when I can get up, I sometimes feel a little better ... A couple of days ago my son really needed help with his homework. His mother was out so I was the only one who could help him. There was something about working alongside him – I just felt a bit better for a while.

Amara: That's interesting. What was it about doing that which made the difference? Do you have any hunches about that?

Dev: (pauses) Maybe I just felt a bit more like my old self. I have always prided myself on being a hands-on dad and helping my son reminded me that despite how bad things have got I can still do things. I've been feeling pretty useless these past weeks, but realising I could help him with his maths ... it showed me that I am still capable of doing things.

Amara: These are important observations you are making. One of the things we know about depression is that it shrinks a person's world. Many people, just like you, feel so weighed down by it that they retreat to bed. But although you go to bed because you feel so bad, lying in bed seems to make things worse, giving you plenty of opportunity to dwell on painful thoughts about yourself, your life and your future. It robs you of doing the things that give you a sense of purpose and success. But when you helped your son, you tapped into that sense of purpose and that felt good.

Dev: It makes sense but there are days where I really just can't get out of bed.

Amara: I know. I am not suggesting that it's straightforward or easy – if it were, you would have fixed things already! But if between us we could think of some ways to help you access more of the feeling that you had when helping your son, would that feel like a step forward?

Dev: Yeah, definitely. I don't know what though ...

Amara: We'll need to think it through, but I have some ideas based on things that have helped other people in the past. Would it be useful if we talked about these and then you can decide what would make most sense to you?

Dev: (sounding a bit more hopeful) I'd like that ...

This transcript highlights information that can provide the basis for guided behaviour change. First, the therapist might introduce a behaviour diary to help build up a picture of what types of activity are associated with both positive and negative changes in Dev's mood, energy or motivation. In this type of diary, the aim is not to provide a comprehensive account of everything that Dev did, thought and felt. Rather, it aims to build up a 'big picture' understanding of the relationship between particular activities and his mood (see Figure 8.1).

Once an activity diary has been completed, therapist and client have important information about how the client is spending their time. Working from the diary example in Figure 8.1, even with just two days completed, Amara can begin to develop hypotheses about what might need to change. For example, she might notice that Dev's typical day offers few opportunities for pleasure and accomplishment and so Amara will likely want to talk with Dev about how to build more of these types of activity back into his life. She might also notice how the occasions when his mood is better coincide with times that he is helping someone he loves (e.g. helping his wife with a problem at work).

Dev is spending a lot of time in bed and during these times his mood worsens. The therapist suspects that when he is in bed, Dev is dwelling on painful ideas about himself, his life and his future – a pattern of cognitive activity known as rumination. So Amara will probably want to find ways to help Dev get out of bed earlier in the day and find new activities in the morning that will engage him in productive activity. These might be pleasurable activities or mastery tasks that afford a sense of accomplishment. Amara might also encourage Dev to introduce some graded exercise into his daily schedule as physical exercise is known to positively impact mood.

Finally, Amara might also seek to recruit Dev's wife to assist him with behavioural activation as this can sometimes increase the effectiveness of therapy for depression (Baucom et al., 2020). Regardless of the method selected, and whether it is implemented by the client or with the additional input of a family member, a key principle is to start with tasks that can be accomplished in the short term and gradually increase the activities according to both difficulty and range so that the client consistently builds on prior successes.

In working with their clients to design a plan of action, it can be useful for therapists to introduce the acronym 'ACE' (available at: www.getselfhelp. co.uk/ace.htm), which stands for:

Achieve: stretching ourselves through work tasks, chores, life admin or study

Connect: with partners, family, friends, community

Enjoy: making time for pleasurable tasks, free time, hobbies

Figure 8.1. Dev's activity diary (a sample of two days)

	Monday	Tuesday	Wednesday	Thursday	Friday	Saturday	Sunday
6–8am	Sleeping	Sleeping					
8–9am	Sleeping	Sleeping					
9–10am	Sleeping	Sleeping					
10–11am	Dozing X	Sleeping					
11–12pm	Got up and had cup of coffee X	Dozing X					
12–1pm	Watched TV X	Lying in bed dozing X					
1–2pm	Watched TV X	Watched TV X					
2–3pm	Watched TV X	Watched TV X					
3–4pm	Watched TV	Went to bed and dozed X					
4–5pm	Cooked son's tea	Watched TV X					
5–6pm	helped son with homework +	Cooked son's tea +					
6–7pm	Talked to wife while she prepared the dinner +	Watched TV					
7–8pm	Dinner with wife	Dinner with wife					
8–9pm	Watched TV with wife	Helped my wife with a problem at work +					
9–10pm	Watched TV with wife	Watched TV with wife					
10–11pm	Watched TV alone	Watched TV alone					
11–12pm	Watched TV alone	Watched TV alone					
12–1am	Watched TV alone	Watched TV alone					

Code key: X = times when mood is particularly low
+ = times when mood is a little better

Helping a client build into their daily schedule at least one activity from each of these three categories can provide a framework for making positive change.

Although in this chapter we have focused on one specific application of guided behaviour change, namely, behavioural activation in the context of depression, it is important to recognise that guided behaviour change is applicable to many areas of life to identify unhelpful patterns, reduce negative behaviours and increase positive behaviours. Both activity diaries as well as the ACE model provide methods for gathering data and designing new ways of behaving that can help a client progress towards the achievement of their goals.

Conclusion

Behavioural methods comprise a rich, diverse and powerful category of intervention that can be tailored to the needs of an individual client to enable change. Although they might appear relatively easy to apply, their skilled use depends on a sound understanding of the nature of the client's difficulties and needs, close collaborative working and careful monitoring as the client experiments with new ways of acting in the pursuit of desired life goals.

In this chapter, we have introduced two broad areas of application: those that have a skills component and those that are focused on guided behaviour change. In addition, behavioural methods can be used in the service of cognitive restructuring – for example, testing out the accuracy of certain cognitions or as means of helping a client confront feared and inappropriately avoided situations. This type of method is the topic of the next chapter.

Reflective Activity: Keeping a diary of how you spend your time

Keep an activity diary for a week, using the type of diary provided in Figure 8.1 (examples are available from Google images). See what you can learn about how you use your time – the balance between pleasure, achievement and chore-related tasks, whether any particular activities are associated with feeling a certain way and whether there are any tasks that you consistently avoid. What do you learn? Are there any changes that would make your typical week feel more rewarding or meaningful to you?

Interested in learning more? Check out …

Trower, P., & Hollin, C. R. (2016). *Handbook of social skills training: Clinical applications and new directions* (Vol. 2). Oxford: Pergamon Press.

McKay, M., Wood, J. C., & Brantley, J. (2007). *The dialectical behavior therapy skills workbook*. Oakland, CA: New Harbinger Publications.

Martell, C. R., Dimidjian, S., & Herman-Dunn, R. (2013). *Behavioural activation for depression: A clinician's guide*. New York: Guilford Press.

NINE

Exposure and Behavioural Experiments

Chapter objectives

By reading this chapter you will be able to:

- Differentiate behavioural interventions used within a behavioural paradigm from those used within a cognitive paradigm
- Understand the rationale and application of exposure and response prevention
- Understand the rationale and application of behavioural experiments
- Appreciate the importance of a collaborative working relationship when using these interventions

Introduction

In contrast to the methods described in the previous chapter where the emphasis was on installing new skills and promoting adaptive behaviour change, this chapter focuses on the use of behaviour methods to help clients confront feared situations (exposure and response prevention) and to test out the accuracy of specific cognitions (behavioural experiments).

Both exposure and response prevention, stemming from the behavioural tradition, and behavioural experiments, stemming from the cognitive tradition, are important interventions for helping clients achieve their goals. They are particularly important in the context of phobias and anxiety disorders but are relevant for a wide variety of emotional difficulties. This chapter introduces these interventions and considers how therapists support clients in engaging with what can be a vital (if at times anxiety-provoking) form of learning.

Exposure and response prevention

Exposure and response prevention (ERP) was originally developed by Meyer (1966). The exposure part of the procedure involves the client intentionally placing themselves in the situation they fear and allowing the anxiety to rise to very high levels. The response prevention part concerns desisting from their usual avoidance, escape or safety-seeking behaviours developed in order to reduce anxiety. Through the use of ERP, clients gradually learn that their anxiety reduces without needing to avoid or escape the feared situation. Increasingly, they become able to tolerate distress without resorting to their coping behaviours and, over time, the anxiety diminishes.

As can be appreciated, implementing ERP requires a sense of assurance and safety that the therapist will manage the situation so that the client is not completely overwhelmed. In the early days, ERP was often conducted in in-patient settings to provide the necessary management and support. Increasingly, alternatives were found to enable ERP to be conducted in out-patient settings, with the client taking more control of the process and the method capitalising on the use of in-vivo (facing the actual feared situation) and imaginal exposure (facing the feared situation in imagination).

One of the areas for which ERP was originally devised was obsessive-compulsive disorder (OCD; Foa, et al., 2012). OCD is a common mental health condition consisting of obsessive thoughts and compulsive behaviours. It affects men, women and children, and while it usually starts in adulthood, early onset around puberty is not uncommon. It can be extremely distressing and interferes significantly with the person's life as the felt need to engage in rituals to relieve the extreme anxiety experienced can consume large amounts of time and prevent engagement in daily activities. For example, the person might excessively wash their hands or feel compelled to check repeatedly that they have locked the front door. Subsequently, they might entertain the thought that perhaps they did not check well enough and need to recheck. OCD was once considered untreatable, but the emergence of ERP changed that widely held belief and ERP has been found to be highly effective as a behavioural intervention to treat the condition (NICE, 2005).

What happens during ERP?

The first phase of ERP consists of assessment and treatment planning. This is a highly collaborative process, aimed at uncovering the stimuli that trigger the obsessive thoughts and distress and identifying external (e.g. situations, objects, people) as well as internal (e.g. thoughts and physiological reactions) factors. Here, the therapist and client undertake a detailed process to describe the content of the obsessions and compulsions and to establish the functional relationship between the two, as described in Chapter 3. A fear hierarchy is established from the least to the most feared situations for subsequent exposure.

In the second phase, therapist and client create repeated opportunities for the client to be exposed to the feared situation without engaging in the compulsive behaviours. Where the behaviour is overt, such as hand washing, the therapist can monitor directly whether the client is refraining. If the client uses ritual thought patterns, the therapist may encourage the use of cognitive tasks designed to interfere with the ritualistic thoughts, such as reciting times tables or counting backwards. Practice might be in-vivo or imaginal depending on the behaviours that need to be confronted. After each exposure session therapist and client review the experience with a focus on what was learned. Active practice between sessions is essential to enable the client to generalise learning to everyday life. As progress is made, the client moves through their fear hierarchy from less to more challenging situations.

The third phase consists of relapse prevention planning, which has several components. It includes agreeing with the client possible early indicators that their symptoms are returning. These are used to remind them to revisit the techniques which have proved helpful and to use them before the symptoms become too strong. This phase can also involve others, such as relatives or friends, who might offer early warnings to the client that they need to act.

It is also the case that difficulties can return without periodic exposure to the feared stimulus. The use of a follow-up session some months after therapy has ended can also be helpful in preventing relapse. Building a narrative for the future is also important so that clients can see themselves as no longer constrained by OCD and can plan how they might like to use the additional time that was formerly taken up by their rituals or other compulsions.

Case study: Jack

Jack, a man in his mid-20s, had developed several checking rituals which had increasingly taken over his life and were now placing his job at risk. One of these was repeatedly checking the gas. He felt the need to check the gas related to intrusive thoughts about being rendered unconscious due to gas poisoning or causing an explosion that would cause harm to others. He was now carrying out multiple mental rituals to try to control the anxiety which was distracting him from doing his job. He was also often late for work because of his checking rituals.

During the assessment and treatment planning phase, Jack learned about OCD and its treatment. His therapist, Sean, worked with him to identify the stimuli that triggered Jack's obsessive thoughts and compulsions. An ABC analysis was undertaken to identify the functional relationships. Checking the gas appeared to begin with the thoughts, "I can't remember turning the gas off. Perhaps I left it on. I need to check again to make sure." Having done so, the thought would occur that, "Perhaps I didn't check properly. Better to be safe than sorry." This would lead to further checking.

Jack's anxiety increased as he imagined various disastrous scenarios that could occur because of having left the gas on. He became so anxious that he could not remember if he had checked, or "checked properly". Thus, although the checking reduced the anxiety initially, it quickly increased as Jack struggled to recall precisely what actions he had, and had not, taken.

Sean encouraged Jack to give himself permission to check, but only once. This procedure contained some important steps. First, when he felt the urge to check, he told himself, "I will check but not for 60 seconds". This break between the urge and the action started to bring the compulsion under his control. With that control in place he then approached the gas taps and stated to himself, "I am now going to check the taps, and this is me taking the steps to properly check". Having checked, he then stated to himself, "I have seen myself check. The gas is now properly turned off and is safe." Thus, Jack had replaced a compulsion to act with a routine (not a ritual) that enabled him to check once but not repeatedly.

If the anxiety returned, he gently but firmly reminded himself that, "I saw myself turn off the tap. There is no need to check again." Using this process, the anxiety over the gas subsided. The process of learning to undertake an analysis of his fears, then finding ways to expose himself to them without engaging in his checking rituals gradually enabled Jack to understand that his fears would subside and that he could overcome them.

To support Jack in relapse prevention, it was agreed that a booster session would be arrange for three months after the end of the therapy.

Behavioural experiments

Unlike ERP, which derives from the behavioural tradition, behavioural experiments are most often associated with the cognitive tradition. Behavioural experiments are planned experiential actions that are undertaken with the therapist or between the sessions (Bennett-Levy et al., 2004). They are a powerful way of helping clients gather information to test the validity of ideas that are central to their concerns.

Behavioural experiments can take different forms. Although they are all based on observation, data-gathering and experimentation, there are two broad categories that a CBT therapist will likely use: (1) those that are discovery-oriented and (2) those that are set up to test specific hypotheses.

Discovery-oriented experiments

Discovery-oriented experiments are used to learn more about a situation where a client lacks information that is important to resolving their difficulties. One commonly used example within this category is the survey method. Surveys can broaden the client's perspective by gathering a sample of opinions about a topic that is relevant to them. For example, in the next case study the therapist, Natalia, helps her client, Chloe, to learn more about her presenting difficulty.

Case study: Chloe

Chloe, a client with body image concerns, believed that, "Men only find women attractive if they are very thin". She initially believed this 100%. Following extensive discussion with her therapist, Natalia, Chloe agreed that it might be helpful to explore this belief further by obtaining a sample of men's criteria for female attractiveness.

The target group of relevance to Chloe was heterosexual men between the ages of 25 and 35. As she felt too embarrassed to approach respondents herself, Natalia agreed to conduct the survey on Chloe's behalf, approaching an initial sample of 15 men (a combination of friends and colleagues who were unknown to Chloe). The questions were collaboratively agreed (see Figure 9.1).

Questions for Survey Participants

What kinds of physical characteristics attract you to a woman?

Is physical appearance the most important thing that attracts you to a woman or are other characteristics important? If so, what are they?

Do you find very thin women attractive?
(On exploration, it was agreed that as this was a subjective and relative term, Chloe would select from the internet an image that reflected her definition of a 'very thin woman' which formed the basis for the final survey question:)

How would you describe the woman in the picture?

1. Very attractive and desirable
2. Moderately attractive and desirable
3. Neutral/neither attractive nor unattractive
4. Moderately unattractive and undesirable
5. Very unattractive and undesirable

Figure 9.1.   Survey to discover what heterosexual men find attractive in a woman

Natalia diligently recorded the responses provided. The outcome of the survey surprised Chloe considerably. The men surveyed reported a wide variety of differing characteristics that they found attractive in a female. None of them spontaneously mentioned thinness as a necessary condition for attraction, although some described being drawn to women who were slim or athletic. Of the 15 men approached, 14 found the image of the very thin woman that the client had selected to be "very unattractive and undesirable".

Having had an opportunity to reflect on the data obtained, Chloe's belief in her target cognition that "Men only find women attractive if they are very thin" reduced from 100% to 70%. Of course, the survey did not address the totality of her problems, but it offered a new perspective on the relationship between thinness and attractiveness that could form the basis of further exploration.

In summary, then, when developing surveys, it is important to:

• Design them collaboratively
• Ensure that the survey questions are constructed carefully so that any responses obtained will have implications for the client's initial perspective
• Identify who will gather the survey responses (therapist, client or both)

- Establish who is the target sample (e.g. adults, only men or women, people in a certain age category or of a particular cultural or professional background)
- Agree how many respondents will be approached in order to obtain a meaningful response to the area of interest

Experiments to test specific hypothesis

Hypothesis-testing experiments are used if a client is making a specific prediction or holds a belief that can be explicitly tested. Here, rather than adopting an open, discovery-oriented mindset, the question to be investigated is clear and focused. These types of experiment are particularly useful for discovering:

- Whether a catastrophic outcome actually occurs (e.g. if a client does in fact have a stroke when they have a panic attack)
- Whether the outcome that the client fears happens but is not as bad as predicted (e.g. a client with social anxiety may, as he fears, stumble on some of his words during a work presentation but is not ridiculed by colleagues as a result)
- How safety-seeking behaviours might be maintaining the problem (e.g. how attempting to suppress intrusive thoughts in the context of OCD might actually increase their frequency and intensity)
- The consequences of reducing or dropping a safety-seeking behaviour (e.g. how reducing the number of times that a health-anxious client checks her breasts for lumps from five times a day to every second day might reduce the frequency of intrusive thoughts about cancer)
- The implications of living life according to a new idea or rule, which we explored in Chapter 6

In conducting a behavioural experiment, clients are typically encouraged to keep a record of their findings, an example of which is included in Figure 9.2.

Date	Situation in which I am conducting the experiment	Prediction: What exactly do I think will happen? How likely do I believe that this will happen 0–100%?	Experiment: How specifically will I test the prediction?	Outcome: What actually happened?	Learning: What did I discover? To what extent was my prediction confirmed?

Figure 9.2.   A behavioural experiment record form

In order to gain the most from the experience, Butler et al. (2008) suggest that, following the experiment, the therapist encourages the client to identify what they learned, how they make sense of the outcome of the experiment, what new information or novel perspectives the outcome suggests, and what this means for the client's original prediction. It is also helpful to consider what implications the outcome of the experiment has for how the client approaches similar situations in the future and what next steps (including further experiments) might now be indicated.

Behavioural experiments follow the scientific principle of making a clear prediction, rating belief in that prediction, testing the prediction, observing the outcome and re-rating the consequences. Thus, the steps involved are typically as follows:

1. Specify the target cognition.
2. Specify the alternative, non-catastrophic cognition.
3. Make a clear prediction.
4. Agree the method to be used.
5. Conduct the experiment.
6. Review the results.
7. Review reflection and learning.
8. Re-rate the target cognition.
9. Consider the implications for the client's understanding of their needs and options.

In the case study below, we provide an illustration of how these principles would be implemented in a case of low mood.

Case study: Erik

Erik was a successful 35-year-old man who had been selected for a placement at the international office of his organisation alongside completing a Master of Science degree. The organisation was interested in exploring the impact of burnout on staff working in high-pressure situations.

On starting his research, Erik began to see conflicts emerging between the demands of the university where he was studying and those of the organisation; while the university sought clear and robust evidence, the organisation was interested in results from which they could learn but which also presented them in a good light. Attempting to navigate these competing priorities led Erik to become increasingly concerned that he was seen as failing by his academic supervisor and disappointing the organisation. Doubts about his own capability intensified and his mood began to deteriorate.

While he continued to function at work, he thought that it was only a matter of time before his 'failure' would be discovered and that he would lose his job.

To prevent being exposed as incompetent, Erik began to avoid engaging with the more challenging aspects of his project and started cancelling meetings with his academic supervisor. He was aware that these short-term attempts at managing his anxiety were simply deferring the problem rather than addressing it.

Erik, together with his therapist, Esther, explored the relationship between his low mood, problematic cognitions and behaviours. One specific cognition appeared to trouble Erik markedly: "If I ask for help my research supervisor will judge me as incompetent for the demands of the project and I shall lose my job." Erik said that he believed this 100%. This became the target cognition for testing.

The next step was to specify an alternative, non-catastrophic cognition. Erik harboured genuine concern about his competence and believed that his livelihood could be at risk. Nonetheless, Esther could not detect any direct evidence to support his catastrophic fear. Following discussion, an alternative perspective was constructed: "Everyone feels vulnerable sometimes. Just because I am struggling does not mean that the project is failing. My academic supervisor is experienced in supervising projects in this type of context and is likely to want to help me." Erik believed this only 50%.

A clear prediction was then identified: "If I tell my supervisor that I am struggling, she will criticise me, distance herself from me and will terminate our working relationship." Erik believed this 90%.

Because Erik perceived the threat to his career to be real, it was agreed that he would first do some background research on other people's experience of his supervisor, which felt less risky in its potential consequences. Through his university, Erik was able to identify several candidates whose research had been supervised by the same individual. He contacted five people and asked about their general experiences of the programme before moving into a discussion about their experience of supervision.

Through tactful questioning, he learned that all the graduates had had positive experiences of the supervisor, who had been constructive and supportive. The graduates also spontaneously disclosed their experiences of how challenging their master's degrees had been and offered Erik advice on how to manage his studies – including the recommendation that he maintain regular contact with his supervisor. This initial experiment reassured Erik greatly. His belief in the original prediction, "If I tell my supervisor that I am struggling, she will criticise me, distance herself from me and will terminate our working relationship," reduced from 100% to only 40%.

Erik then felt ready to take the risk of speaking directly with his supervisor. Having discussed several ways of approaching this situation in therapy, he arranged a tutorial with a view to sharing the extent of his recent struggles. Esther asked him to observe his supervisor's reactions carefully, making a note of any critical comments and whether his supervisor subsequently withdrew from their relationship.

The results of the experiment were illuminating. Although Erik had felt very uncomfortable about disclosing his difficulties, he experienced his supervisor as concerned, attentive and supportive. She revealed that she had wondered why Erik had kept cancelling their meetings but now she understood she suggested that they increase the frequency of contact to ensure that Erik felt supported.

His supervisor further confirmed that she did not doubt his capability for master's level work. Nonetheless, she did have concerns about the viability of the project given that the organisation seemed to want to guide the data to a pre-determined result. As they talked through the context of the project, Erik's supervisor helped him to frame questions that could open up the possibility of a useful conversation with the organisation as to how to devise a worthwhile piece of research.

At this point, Erik's belief in his prediction, "If I tell my supervisor that I am struggling, she will criticise me, distance herself from me and will terminate our working relationship", reduced to 0%. His belief in the original target cognition, "If I ask for help my supervisor will judge me as too weak and incompetent for the demands of the project and I shall lose my job", had also reduced to 0%.

Erik was relieved but also surprised by how inaccurate his target cognition had proved to be. With the aid of Esther, he began to appreciate that his anxieties were being expressed at various levels in the organisation. The conflicts he had been experiencing also appeared to be mirrored in wider issues relating to the culture of the organisation. As it became clear that the doubts were real but had been misinterpreted as personal to him, Erik felt empowered to negotiate with the organisation and his university as to how the research would be conducted.

While the therapy could have ended at that point, Erik was concerned to understand how his mood had deteriorated so rapidly. Therapy then began to focus on his core beliefs (see Chapter 6). It became clear that as a child he had been very clever, much praised in his family for his academic prowess and had only ever experienced success. However, his family was also emotionally distant; anxieties could not be discussed and problems needed to have logical solutions. He began to understand that his core beliefs about himself operated through a narrow lens in which he had to see the world in very logical terms. Faced with overwhelming feelings and deteriorating mood he had no understanding of how to deal with his circumstances. Using his existing intellectual skills had led him down a path of misinterpretation because he was unable to recognise and accept his feelings, ask for help or seek support from those around him – including his supervisor. This realisation led to a new phase of therapy in which the focus was on helping Erik modify some of his core beliefs in order to build a new narrative about himself, his self-worth and his future.

Conclusion

This chapter has presented different ways of approaching fears that reflect the perspectives on emotional distress arising from each of the behavioural principle and the cognitive principle. In the case of ERP, exposure to a feared situation and discovering that the fear subsides enables problems to be overcome. Behavioural experiments also provide a way to confront fears but do so through helping the client test the cognitions associated with patterns of distress and avoidance.

Alongside the cognitive techniques explored in the other chapters, ERP and behavioural experiments are widely used in CBT. Approached with a spirit of discovery rather than a need to prove an outcome, they offer excellent and, at times, transformational learning experiences.

Reflective Activity: Devising next steps for the case studies in this chapter

Choose the case of Chloe or Erik. Based on what you have learned, what other experiments might you devise to test their beliefs? Think through the questions you might ask and the procedure you would use.

If you prefer, reflect on the case of Jack and consider the relapse prevention phase. What might you explore with Jack to help him build a new narrative for himself and his future that is no longer focused on the OCD?

Interested in learning more? Check out …

Foa, E. B., Yadin, E., & Lichner, T. K. (2012). *Exposure and response (ritual) prevention for obsessive-compulsive disorder: Therapist guide* (2nd ed.). Oxford: Oxford University Press.

Bennett-Levy, J., Butler, G., Fennell, M., Hackmann, A., Mueller, M., & Westbrook, D. (2004). *Oxford guide to behavioural experiments in cognitive therapy*. Oxford: Oxford University Press.

Part III
Using CBT in Therapy and Beyond

TEN

Formulation in Cognitive Behaviour Therapy

Chapter objectives

By reading this chapter you will be able to:

- Understand why formulation is central to CBT
- Understand how a CBT therapist makes sense of a client's needs using cognitive and behavioural concepts
- Describe the different types and levels of formulation commonly used in CBT

Introduction

So far in this book, you have been introduced to some of the main principles and methods that commonly feature in CBT practice. In this chapter we explore how a therapist synthesises those principles and methods with the client's story in order to decide upon an intervention plan. First, we describe what is meant by the term 'formulation' and why this is deemed to be central to CBT. We then describe the different types of formulation which a CBT therapist might use to make sense of a client's needs. Finally, to bring these to life, we present a case study of how a formulation might be developed at different levels as information about the client's needs is collected over time.

What is formulation?

A formulation is a psychologically-informed explanation of the client's concerns that has implications for change (Corrie & Lane, 2010). The aim of a formulation is to devise a personalised theory of a client's problem that can account for why they are experiencing a particular problem at a particular point in their lives. This personalised theory also needs to illuminate potential ways forward through identifying aspects of cognition, behaviour and environment that are amenable to change. To arrive at this explanatory account, a formulation draws together theory, research and practice and, as such, synthesises the client's story with relevant cognitive and behavioural principles.

Why is formulation important?

Formulation is widely regarded as being central to effective CBT (J. S. Beck, 2011; Bruch, 2015; Corrie et al., 2016) and for good reason. Underpinning practice with a formulation provides numerous benefits, including:

- Helping build a comprehensive picture of a client's needs
- Making links between apparently disparate problems that have implications for the approach to change that is adopted
- Locating the client's difficulties in the context of their personal history and life circumstances
- Promoting a sense of hope for the client (and sometimes the therapist) that the client's difficulties have occurred for a reason and can be understood and addressed
- Synthesising multiple sources of information (e.g. clinical interview, self-report measures, observations, reports from family members) into a coherent account

- Making connections between cognitions, emotions, physical reactions, behaviours and environmental factors
- Clarifying relevant areas for exploration and hypothesis-testing
- Aiding the identification of priorities and goals for therapy
- Assisting with intervention planning and decision-making about which CBT techniques to use
- Predicting and responding to obstacles to change
- Making sense of a client's response to therapy over time
- Thinking creatively about lack of progress

Approaches to CBT formulation

Just as CBT is not a single, unified field, there is no single, right way to approach the task of formulation. For example, therapists who are behaviourally-oriented will typically use functional analysis, seeking to understand patterns of stimulus (A), behaviour (B) and consequence (C). In contrast, therapists who are cognitively-oriented will privilege patterns of thinking and information-processing, as well as thoughts, assumptions and beliefs that impact our emotional experience and actions in the world.

Moreover, while some approaches adopt a generic approach, seeking to help a client create links between situation, emotion, thought and behaviour (e.g. Greenberger & Padesky, 2015), other formulations are disorder-specific, providing a framework for making sense of common mental health problems that are grounded in existing CBT theory and research. It is also common practice to develop a longitudinal formulation in which the client's needs can be located within their personal, social and cultural history, which can be useful where a client has concerns across multiple life areas rather than any specific clinical disorder.

In their review of the different ways in which formulation can be approached, Corrie et al. (2016) highlight three different levels of case formulation, drawing on the earlier work of Persons and Davidson (2010). These are:

1. Formulation at the level of the situation.
2. Formulation at the level of the problem.
3. Formulation at the level of the case.

Each of these levels guides the focus of the exploration towards gathering specific types of information. As these levels illustrate how CBT therapists would apply the principles and concepts introduced in the previous chapters, we describe these below before illustrating how they might look in practice.

1. Formulation at the level of the situation

A formulation at the situation level focuses on a client's experiences and responses in a specific situation at a particular point in time. Here, the focus is on eliciting the micro-level factors that are supporting or inhibiting the client's emotions, physical sensations and cognitions, and how these relate to any resulting behaviour or other consequences.

Formulating at the level of the situation is likely to be initiated by the therapist asking the client to provide a recent, specific example of the problem. The aim is to understand in detail the distressing emotions and sensations that illustrate the problem in action as well as eliciting negative automatic thoughts (see Chapters 2 and 5) and approaches to coping that may represent a form of avoidance or other safety-seeking behaviours (Chapter 3).

2. Formulation at the level of the problem

A formulation at the problem level is concerned with understanding the factors that are implicated in similar types of reaction across situations. Each situation represents one instance of a problematic pattern in the client's life more broadly. Hence, it will be useful to look beyond any specific, recent example in order to understand underlying patterns that could be important to address.

Working at the level of the problem is also where therapists will draw on disorder-specific formulations to guide their thinking. Thus, in compiling a list of a client's concerns, it may become apparent that the client is in fact reporting a set of difficulties consistent with diagnostic criteria for a disorder such as depression, generalised anxiety disorder or post-traumatic stress disorder. This understanding can then guide the therapist to those CBT principles, models and methods that are most likely to be relevant to the client's needs.

3. Formulation at the level of the case

There will be occasions when developing a broader understanding of the client's background and personal, educational and professional history is necessary to devise an intervention that is optimally effective. Here, the aim is to understand the client's story, taking account of both proximal and distal factors.

At the case level, areas of interest include (1) factors that have predisposed the client to the problem/s of concern, (2) factors that have precipitated the areas of concern, (3) factors that have helped maintain the problem, and (4) any protective factors that have lessened the impact or that might be harnessed in order to facilitate change (Kuyken et al., 2009).

The therapist will also seek to create links between the overt difficulties with which a client is presenting and any underlying psychological mechanisms that are driving them (Persons, 2012) as well as any under- and over-developed methods of coping. These would include attending to enduring cognitions, such as core beliefs and assumptions (Chapter 6), as well as any reasoning biases (Chapter 2) and patterns of behaviour, such as avoidance (Chapter 3).

Thus, formulating at the level of the case may involve integrating several situation or problem level formulations and is concerned with locating the difficulties the client is experiencing within a larger personal, professional and social context.

To illustrate how these different levels of formulation might look in practice, the next case study describes how Daan, a CBT therapist, works with Suma, a client who is experiencing difficulties with anxiety in the context of work-related social interactions.

Case study: Suma

Suma presented for help with low mood and "feeling stressed". On further exploration during the initial consultation, she explained that "feeling stressed" was exclusive to social situations and that she was feeling low because of her difficulties interacting with others.

Suma was training to be a secondary school teacher and at the age of 22 had realised that what she had initially dismissed as youthful shyness was beginning to handicap her professional choices. At the time of her self-referral, things had become so difficult that she was considering leaving her teacher training.

Although Suma could largely manage the classroom setting, she struggled with the necessary observations by senior colleagues. Moreover, informal encounters with colleagues in the staff room, as well as staff meetings and contact with colleagues during extra-curricular activities, proved excruciating. Suma's aim for therapy was to "become more confident" in her interactions with colleagues so that she could successfully complete her training and fulfil her vocational aspiration of becoming a qualified teacher.

The process of formulation began by constructing a problem list of the difficulties that Suma was experiencing, which she described as follows:

- Feeling very anxious in social situations involving colleagues
- Blushing in the presence of colleagues
- Sweating in the presence of colleagues
- Feeling "weird and spaced out" when talking to senior colleagues
- Stuttering when talking to colleagues
- Avoiding informal encounters with colleagues wherever possible
- Low mood

Daan noted that despite her fears, Suma did not particularly blush in his presence nor was there any evidence of stuttering or sweating. However, her eye contact was poor and Daan noted that Suma was wearing unusually heavy make-up.

Formulation at the level of the situation

In order to develop a formulation at the level of situation, Daan asked Suma to "talk him through a recent incident" where she had experienced the problem so that they could develop an understanding of what had precipitated the problem, what specific emotions, sensations and cognitions were present during the event and how Suma had responded to what was occurring.

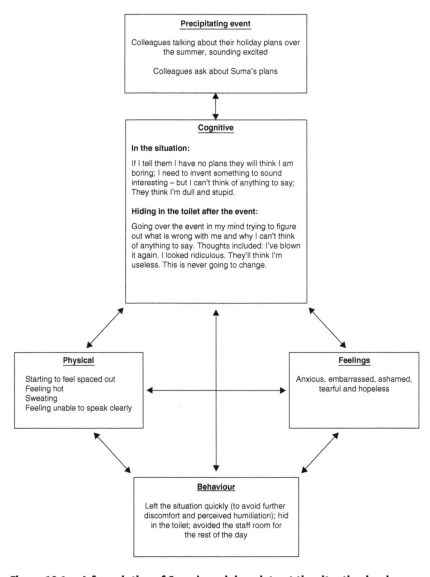

Figure 10.1.   A formulation of Suma's social anxiety at the situation level

Suma described a situation in which she was in the staff room during a lunch break with two of her qualified colleagues. They were talking about their holiday plans at the end of term and asked Suma what she had planned. Suma recalled immediately feeling anxious as she had no plans to go away and would be spending the summer with her family at home. She recalled thinking, "They'll think I am boring if I tell them the truth. I'd better make something up to sound interesting". When she could not think of anything to say, she experienced herself as blushing and stuttering. She quickly excused herself, locked herself in the toilet and tried to calm herself while ruminating on how her colleagues would have been judging her for "being inadequate".

Daan and Suma created a visual representation of this process, as shown in Figure 10.1.

Formulation at the level of the problem

At their first meeting, and in light of the presenting concerns and problem list, Daan asked Suma to complete some self-report measures. Her results revealed that she was experiencing moderately high levels of low mood and moderately high levels of anxiety. Her score profile placed her within the clinically significant range for social anxiety disorder.

Daan's working hypothesis was that Suma's difficulties were consistent with a presentation of social anxiety disorder and the recent, situation-specific examples that they reviewed together appeared to support this hypothesis. Drawing on his knowledge of disorder-specific models, Daan described how social anxiety is believed to be underpinned by a fear of negative evaluation – an idea with which Suma readily concurred. Because of this fear, a person is highly sensitive to any potential signs of criticism and will tend to interpret neutral or ambiguous reactions as signs of disapproval. Suma was able to give several examples of how this idea applied to her and worked with Daan to identify the sequence of relevant cognitions, emotions and sensations in each case, as illustrated in Figures 10.2 and 10.3.

Once she had escaped to safety, Suma would repeatedly go over what had happened. This would give rise to cognitions such as, "They think I'm ridiculous. I *am* ridiculous. What's the matter with me? I'm not like other people. This is hopeless." She would then feel very low and contemplate leaving the profession.

Given these processes, Daan asked Suma how she had managed to cope with the problem at the time it was happening. Through Daan's use of guided discovery, Suma began to appreciate how her well-intentioned use of counter-productive safety-seeking strategies, while reducing her experience of distress in the moment, could be maintaining her social anxiety over the longer term. For example, rehearsing what she would say before speaking, in an attempt to come across as fluent in her speech, had the unintended consequence of inhibiting effective listening and spontaneity. Likewise, wearing heavy make-up to hide her blushing resulted in a slightly unusual appearance that Daan thought could lead people to take a second glance at her and mark her out as 'different'.

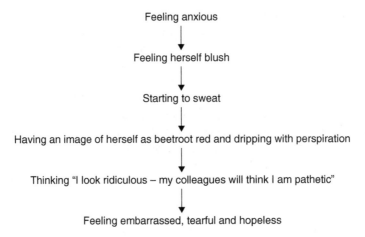

Figure 10.2.   Formulation at the problem level: sequence 1

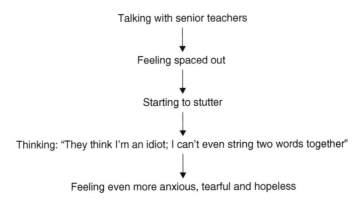

Figure 10.3.   Formulation at the problem level: sequence 2

An additional idea to which her therapist introduced Suma was how the attention of socially anxious people becomes very self-focused during social interactions. According to Clark and Wells (1995), when individuals who are socially anxious believe that they are at risk of negative evaluation, they move their attention inwards, engaging in detailed self-monitoring of their performance. This self-monitoring leads to a greater and unhelpful awareness of internal information (e.g. thoughts, feelings and physical sensations) which is used to infer how the self appears to others and how others will be judging them; that is, feeling anxious is equated with looking anxious, and feeling hot is equated with extreme sweating that is visible to those around them. Suma strongly identified with these theoretically-informed ideas. She also disclosed another well-described phenomenon for socially anxious individuals – namely, images of herself as viewed from an observer's perspective. From what she described, these images seemed distorted in a negative way and inconsistent with Daan's visual impression of her, and therefore suggested that Suma had some maladaptive imagery that could be an important target of intervention.

Formulation at the level of the case

Having worked with Daan to formulate her difficulties at the level of situation and problem, Suma started to feel more optimistic that her difficulties could potentially be understood and managed. A disorder-specific model that had been developed by CBT scholars implied that other people also experienced social anxiety. This helped her feel less alone. However, from the information that she had provided about her background, her therapist deemed it useful to work with Suma to locate her current challenges within a longitudinal formulation that encompassed predisposing factors from her personal history.

Suma had been a shy, quietly industrious child who had often felt overshadowed by her three older, more gregarious siblings. She came from a high-achieving, British-Asian family that demanded the best and where educational achievement was prized above all else. In her family, respect for hierarchy was emphasised and, over time, she had learned the importance of seeking to please high-status people.

In her family of origin, vulnerability was considered a sign of weakness. She had an aunt who suffered from depression and periodically required in-patient treatment, which was viewed negatively within the family; the aunt was never mentioned. More generally, feelings were rarely talked about at home and Suma had learned to deal with any emotional discomfort or needs by simply ignoring them or distracting herself away from them.

Her experiences at school had been based on a sense of being driven to succeed and a lack of popularity with her peers, who labelled her "a swot". She was bullied over several years for her studious approach and cultural background but never felt able to disclose what was happening to her as she believed that to do so would be a sign of weakness.

As they explored these factors, Daan and Suma began to develop a formulation that incorporated the following core beliefs:

- I am different (in a bad way)
- I am weak
- People don't like me
- I am not as good as others

The rules and standards that had emerged from these core beliefs included:

- I should keep my views to myself otherwise people will judge me badly
- I should always excel or I'll let my parents down and be seen as a failure

- If I feel anxious it means I am weak (and if people see I am weak they will reject me)
- It is terrible if someone doesn't like me
- If I keep my head down, people will leave me alone

Suma had managed her early experiences of being bullied by withdrawing emotionally and socially and throwing herself into her schoolwork, which fitted with her parents' beliefs about the pivotal importance of working hard at school. Although this had helped limit her distress at the time, Daan hypothesised that this method of self-protection had become embedded at the expense of developing other life skills; that is, her use of avoidant methods of coping had become an over-developed strategy for managing challenging situations. On further exploration, it appeared that Suma had not had opportunities for developing the psychological problem-solving and assertiveness skills that would be necessary to navigate her circumstances effectively.

Daan also hypothesised that Suma had a limited understanding of emotions in that she struggled to identify, label, differentiate and manage different emotional states. She did not appear to know how to self-soothe during times of distress or engage in other methods of mood management other than distraction. This made sense in the context of her family, where feelings had rarely been talked about and were regarded with suspicion.

Finally, Daan noted that while Suma was able to report her perceived deficits, she struggled to identify her strengths and accomplishments, of which there were many. He introduced Suma to the idea of reasoning biases, including discounting positives, exaggerating negatives and, in the context of social situations, mind reading (Chapter 2). They also considered relevant protective factors that could be harnessed to help Suma make the changes in her life that she wished to see.

What might Daan have done next?

It is important to note that the levels of formulation outlined above are not mutually exclusive. In practice, therapists typically draw on all three but may introduce them at different stages. While a situation-specific formulation is typically used early on, formulation at the level of the case often takes longer and reflects the accumulation of information about a client and their historical and current context over time. Although different in emphasis, each of these levels provides a therapist with choices as to how to intervene. For example, at the situation level, Daan might ask Suma to keep a diary of challenging situations as the basis for an ABC analysis (Chapter 3). This could reveal sequences across situations of the kind illustrated above. He might then help Suma identify what could be done differently: for example, dealing with physical tension by learning controlled breathing techniques or modifying unhelpful cognitions through use of thought records (Chapter 5) as well as modifying her maladaptive coping behaviours.

Alternatively, Daan might use the situation-specific examples to confirm a working hypothesis that Suma is experiencing social anxiety disorder and move directly into working at the level of the problem. Here, he would be informed by disorder-specific thinking about how to help Suma modify self-focused attention and would likely develop a series of behavioural experiments to test her catastrophic predictions and the consequences of changing her usual patterns of coping (e.g. avoiding eye contact and wearing heavy make-up). Gaining objective feedback on her social performance through video feedback would also be a likely strategy in line with current guidance on how to work with social anxiety.

At the level of the case, Daan might aim to work with some of Suma's rules for living and core beliefs (Chapter 6). He might consider helping her develop skills in key areas, including assertiveness, social skills (if these were identified as deficient in some way) and emotion regulation (Chapter 8). The formulation at the case level suggested these areas as under-developed methods of coping that could provide an alternative to her currently dominant avoidant methods of coping. There might also be a need to re-examine her sense of being "different" in the context of her experiences of having been bullied – both for her diligent approach to her studies and because of her cultural background.

Formulation as a complex skill

Formulation is perhaps one of the most complex and sophisticated tasks that a CBT therapist undertakes. As a result, it takes time to learn and is a skill that is best acquired through the guidance and support of a supervisor.

As a vehicle for making sense of a client's difficulties and needs, formulation relies upon the effective use of a range of generic as well as CBT-specific skills. These include generating and testing relevant hypotheses, gathering and interpreting data from a number of sources (e.g. the client's story, self-report measures, the therapist's observations), a knowledge of relevant theory and research and an informed understanding of the client's social, economic and cultural context and how these inform the client's experience. For these reasons, formulation does not lend itself to operationalisation and measurement in the way that is perhaps characteristic of other components of CBT practice. Yet where it is done effectively and collaboratively, a formulation brings to the therapy a means for therapist and client to devise an action plan that makes sense to both parties, and which incorporates the factors that are amenable to change.

Conclusion

This chapter has introduced the place of formulation within CBT. Although it can take several forms, in broad terms a formulation is the means through which clients can organise their understanding of their experiences and therapists can bring fresh perspectives to highlight potential avenues for change.

As illustrated through the case of Suma, regardless of the approach adopted, a formulation is always informed by relevant theoretical constructs, principles and contemporary thinking about how best to work with specific presentations. Nonetheless, even when they are available, it is never the case that a client is 'fitted' to an existing model. Clients' needs do not always present as clearly defined or take the form of single life problems for which our CBT methods offer neat prescriptions. Hence therapists need to avoid the trap of foreclosing the emerging narrative by engaging fully with the client's story. Only then is it possible to work together to devise an effective plan for change.

Reflective Activity: Applying formulation to your own life

Try creating a formulation of your life up to a specific point or, if you prefer, an account of where you are in your career as of today.
  Consider:

- Predisposing factors: what influences from the past were important in getting you to this point? What beliefs and attitudes from the past are still influencing you today?
- Precipitating factors: how do you feel right now having thought about the past? Describe what you immediately thought and felt as you completed the task. Then consider what thoughts are implicated in how you are feeling right now.
- Perpetuating factors: do you wish to continue in the same way? If you are feeling positive, what might you do to reinforce (increase) and maintain its occurrence? If you are feeling negative, what might you do to decrease that feeling based on the ideas presented in this book?
- Protective factors: what influences can you draw upon to protect against any problems? What resources do you have available to you – personal and environmental – that you can harness to support you in your endeavours?

Now rewrite your formulation considering your responses to the above and see if you can devise a plan to enhance your journey towards where you want to be.

Interested in learning more? Check out ...

Bruch, M. (2015). *Beyond diagnosis: Case formulation in cognitive behavioural therapy* (2nd ed.). Chichester, UK: Wiley Blackwell. NB: This book introduces the origins of individualised case formulation and provides an illustrative series of case studies in current practice.

Corrie, S., Townend, M. J., & Cockx, A. (2016). *Assessment and case formulation in cognitive behavioural therapy* (2nd ed.). London: SAGE. NB: This book provides a detailed account of how to craft CBT formulations generically and for different types of presenting problems.

Corrie, S., & Lane, D. A. (2010). *Constructing stories, telling tales: A guide to formulation in applied psychology.* London: Karnac. NB: This book explores the concept of formulation more broadly and draws on insights from psychology and the arts.

ELEVEN

Future Directions for Cognitive Behaviour Therapy

Chapter objectives

By reading this chapter you will be able to:

- Better understand the challenges facing our global physical and mental health needs and have some ideas as to how CBT might be part of an effective response to these challenges
- Appreciate how a number of initiatives in CBT have come about through an alliance with the medical model
- Describe current challenges – from within CBT and beyond – that are likely to influence how the field evolves

Introduction

The principal aim of this book has been to provide an introduction to the field of CBT to help you understand more about its origins and development and how CBT is currently practised. But what of the future? Or, put slightly differently, what might be needed of CBT in the future and how might its models, methods and techniques have to evolve to meet these needs?

In this final chapter, we share some thoughts about the challenges and opportunities that will likely face CBT in the years ahead. We declare at the outset that some of the perspectives we present sit firmly outside any currently authorised version of CBT and also relate to other psychologically-informed interventions. Nonetheless, remaining true to the spirit of innovation that has always characterised the field, we offer these perspectives as potentially valuable avenues for the advancement of theory, research, practice and models of delivery in a world which promises a future profoundly different from the past.

Equipping ourselves for the world of tomorrow: identifying the challenge

Despite significant advancements in our understanding of many physical and mental health conditions, the human race is a long way from flourishing. Indeed, the available statistics paint a deeply concerning picture about our collective health and well-being. For example, the World Health Organisation (WHO) has reported that approximately 450 million people globally are living with a mental health problem (WHO, 2001). In England, common mental health problems are believed to affect at least one in six adults (McManus et al., 2016) and 20% of older adults (WHO, 2019).[1] Approximately 20% of adolescents experience a mental health problem in any given year (WHO, 2003), with clinically diagnosable problems also affecting 10% of children aged 5–16 (Green et al., 2005). For good reason then, mental health problems have been identified as one of the main disease burdens worldwide (Vos et al., 2015).

Our physical health is also a cause for concern. The incidence of long-term health conditions is rising, as is multimorbidity: that is, individuals living with more than one medical condition. For example, in the UK alone it is estimated that approximately 15 million people are now living with a long-term health condition which will require ongoing management (The King's Fund, 2020). This has significant implications for how health services are delivered. NHS England (2014) has stated that treating and managing long-term conditions is now a central focus of NHS services, which must reconsider their priorities as well as how their staff are trained to meet those priorities. In summary, it would seem reasonable to conclude that alongside the expansion of psychological services, a more radical reconsideration is needed of how CBT might be delivered and shared. This entails a reconceptualisation of the challenges ahead and how, as a community, we should respond.

Equipping ourselves for the world of tomorrow: conceptualising the challenge

It is self-evident that life today is quite different from life in the 20th century. Collectively, we find ourselves confronting unprecedented challenges to our global well-being, societal infrastructures and economies. The clients of CBT services, alongside the professionals who support them, are having to navigate an increasingly volatile, uncertain, complex and ambiguous world (Barber, 1992), where contexts are more complex, needs are harder to define and measure, and outcomes are less predictable.

The importance of finding new ways of working effectively within contexts that serve up paradox and uncertainty rather than trying to eliminate or otherwise manage these realities is now widely recognised. For example, in the context of understanding and enabling effective organisational leadership, complexity theorists (e.g. Stacey 2010; Boulton et al., 2015) have argued that rather than attempting to envision and predict the future, leaders need an ability to cultivate the conditions that allow creative solutions to emerge from the interactions of the agents within the organisation. A similar argument has been made within the field of coaching (Cavanagh & Lane, 2012; Kovacs & Corrie, 2017).

One useful response to conceptualising the challenges currently faced by humankind is the concept of the wicked problem. The term 'wicked problem' was originally coined by Rittel and Webber (1973) but has considerable contemporary relevance. More recently, in continuing this line of scholarly enquiry, Brown et al. (2010) have characterised a wicked problem as:

> ...a complex issue that defies complete definition, for which there can be no final solution, since any resolution generates further issues, and where solutions are not true or false or good or bad, but the best that can be done at the time. (Brown et al., 2010: 4)

Wicked problems acquire their complexity in part because they are embedded within the very societies that generate them. In consequence, any solutions will entail a re-evaluation of societal structures, processes, practices and traditions, and will require changes in how its members act. Examples of wicked problems include climate change, how to develop sustainable resources as the global population increases, immigration, terrorism, gang warfare, poverty, and data security and privacy in an online world. They also include the mental health needs facing the population, the rise of chronic health conditions and the onset of global pandemics.

It is important to note that use of the term 'wicked' does not imply that the issue itself is evil in any moral sense. Rather, it denotes a particular kind of challenge whose complexity evades our existing problem-solving strategies and which can create a sense of being "... locked in an endless spiral from which there is no escape" (Brown et al., 2010: 3). Thus, viewed through the lens of the wicked problem, it is unlikely that sustainable solutions to our health and well-being needs can come from increasing existing resources alone. Rather, staying healthy in the 21st century will require new forms of thinking and learning from multiple disciplines. It is our belief that CBT can play a central role in meeting our collective physical and emotional well-being needs in this context.

Equipping ourselves for the world of tomorrow: responding to the challenge

In considering what might be needed of CBT in the future and how its models and methods of practice would have to evolve to address it, we identify three levels where we believe that CBT can add value. These are: (1) the changing needs of clients; (2) the emerging needs of the workforce; and (3) embedding or 'seeding' CBT within wider community and social systems. We consider each of these in turn, identifying what we would see as some important questions for progressing the development of CBT at each of these levels.

1. Responding to the changing needs of clients

Traditionally in CBT, the dominant model for the treatment of psychological difficulties and disorders has, in many cases, been working exclusively with the client who is identified as needing help. The emphasis on developing interventions to address client psychopathology stems from the influence of the medical model, whereby the distressed individual is diagnosed with a disorder which is then treated, where possible, through the delivery of an empirically-supported intervention. CBT has a very well-established history for working at this level and has provided the field with protocols, principles and methods that have extended the reach of CBT to an increasingly diverse range of client issues. When David et al. (2018: 1) refer to CBT as the "current gold standard of psychotherapy", it is this level of contribution to which they are referring. Moreover, where funding for psychological therapies is limited, and where commissioners of services have to make difficult decisions about spending priorities, the assurance of an intervention that is empirically-supported is appealing and fits well with the evidence-based health care agenda that is dominant in current health care systems.

The client, of course, does not just refer to an individual, and facilitating change often includes others involved in the client's life, such as a life partner, parent, family system or teacher. Moreover, from within the field itself, there have been challenges to the tendency of CBT to work with the client apart from the systems in which they are embedded. Baucom et al. (2018), for example, have argued convincingly for the value of addressing psychopathology through CBT couple-focused interventions. Their principle-driven rather than protocol-driven approach offers what they propose is a much-needed paradigm shift in how psychological difficulties are conceptualised and treated. Specifically, they claim that CBT needs to develop a broader interpersonal perspective which reflects the interdependence that is a hallmark of healthy adult functioning. One development, then, is how the field can develop criteria to determine when CBT is most usefully delivered to the individual client and when it includes others within the client's system.

A further development for the future is reflected in the growing number of CBT therapies that have grappled with knowing how and when to build resilience in our clients as opposed to treating psychopathology. Historically, the emphasis of the methods discussed in the previous chapters has reflected a desire to equip individuals with ways of responding to problems of living that can address future challenges in addition to current ones. However, other approaches within the family of CBT therapies have sought to extend this contribution. For example, and as identified in Chapter 1, many of the so-called third wave approaches are concerned primarily with helping individuals develop psychological processes that can enable well-being rather than aiming for symptom reduction.

One example of working with strengths is Positive CBT (Bannink, 2012). The aim of Positive CBT is to synthesise the contributions of CBT, solution-focused approaches and positive psychology to empower a client in building success. In offering a radically new perspective on the aims and methods of therapy, Positive CBT represents a challenge to problem-focused ways of working grounded in the medical model, where the nature of the problem needs to be diagnosed before an appropriate treatment can be identified. By focusing not on clients' difficulties and limitations but on their capabilities, strengths and resources, the approach claims to facilitate improved well-being and quality of life alongside enhanced functioning at the personal, interpersonal and social levels.

Together, the carefully developed and empirically validated methods that target psychopathology and other problems of living combined with the emergent strengths-based approaches aimed at promoting well-being create a powerful offering for our turbulent times.

Questions for theory, research and practice arising from this level include:

- Which forms of client difficulty will need to be a priority focus for the development of new treatment protocols?
- When should CBT focus on treating psychopathology and when should it focus on building strengths?
- What resources and capabilities are needed to equip individuals for the demands and challenges of the modern world?
- What does resilience look like when conceptualised within a CBT framework?

2. Responding to the emerging needs of the workforce

Staff well-being is a critical component of effective and responsive CBT services. In professional services more widely, there is growing recognition of the support needs of workers and organisations, particularly for those dealing with high levels of stress. This would include those employed in social work, the emergency services, the police, air traffic control and health and social care professionals who, as a consequence of their work, can experience the impact of secondary exposure to trauma and are prone to compassion fatigue and burnout (Tehrani, 2011). These phenomena are just as relevant to CBT therapists and require both responsive and preventative action. Interesting studies are emerging that suggest that fostering mindfulness and resilience can positively impact client outcomes (Pereira et al., 2017) and the nature and role of personal practices adopted by CBT therapists during training have been studied by Bennett-Levy (2019). However, a robust understanding of how to support the resilience of the CBT workforce is yet to be established. As we would see it, this is a priority area for research and practice, especially given the ongoing expansion of services delivering CBT interventions through, for example, the IAPT initiative.

The implementation of the IAPT programme (Department of Health, 2008) has resulted in a radical change to the way in which psychological interventions generally and CBT specifically are delivered within primary care services. The IAPT programme is underpinned by the principles of (1) offering evidence-based psychological treatments at the appropriate dose, (2) ensuring that these interventions are delivered by a workforce that is trained and supervised to ensure high-quality care and fidelity to NICE guidance, and (3) routine outcome monitoring. Since its introduction, this model of service delivery has been extended to include those with long-term conditions, children and young people and couple-based interventions, as well as focusing on increasing access to, and uptake by, older people and black, Asian and minority ethnic (BAME) populations (see National Collaborating Centre for Mental Health, 2019).

A consequence of the IAPT initiative has been the creation of an entirely new and expanding CBT workforce. For example, in the *NHS Five Year Forward Review* for Mental Health, NHS England (2014) confirmed its commitment to expanding IAPT services to enable at least 1.5 million adults to access psychological treatments each year. This requires a significant increase in the number of those qualified to deliver these interventions. However, relatively little is known about this new workforce, including what they need to sustain themselves in terms of opportunities for learning and development, and methods of self-care that would empower them to deliver their best work.

In this climate of uncertainty and change, other groups are also moving into the mental health and well-being arena. In certain cases, these groups can bring valuable and different expertise from fields such as occupational health, human resource well-being and coaching. Here, they are not acting as therapists but can facilitate change in the broader areas of a client's life that have not traditionally been the province of therapists (Tehrani & Lane, in press). Nonetheless, other professional groups, such as coaches, are starting to lay claim to forms of expertise previously delivered by those having completed a core mental health training (see for example, Wolever et al.'s (2013) systematic review of the literature on health and wellness coaching and the emerging specialism of mental health coaching reviewed by Corrie and Parsons (in press)). Although such developments require careful judgements about where these types of services can add value as well as how they are supported and regulated, it seems likely that new service offerings delivered by new workforces will continue in the future as public sector services grapple with increasingly intractable financial challenges.

Questions for theory, research and practice arising from this level include:

* Who are the CBT workforces of today and what enables their resilience?
* Who are the CBT workforces of tomorrow and what will enable their resilience? How well equipped are those delivering CBT interventions to respond to the levels of complexity that they encounter in their work settings? What do they need to be better equipped for the challenges of tomorrow?
* What are the well-being needs of the CBT workforce?
* What self-care practices are needed for CBT practitioners of all kinds to remain well, protect themselves from compassion fatigue and burnout, and thrive?

3. Embedding CBT within wider social and community systems

A more radical area of development for CBT comes from considering how its principles and methods might be 'seeded' in our communities and society.

This speaks to the as yet largely untapped potential of CBT as a means of system transformation.

The idea that our psychological knowledge and methods should be used for the purposes of social transformation has long been debated. Indeed, a recognition that the solution to many of the difficulties we encounter lies in a need to change our social institutions was strongly advocated by George Miller in his 1969 Presidential Address to the American Psychological Association. Miller emphasised that in order for psychology to fulfil its potential as a means of promoting human welfare, we need to "give psychology away" (Miller, 1969). Although CBT has always championed the notion of empowerment through offering clients techniques that can help maintain well-being over time, to "give away" CBT in the sense that Miller described argues for a more radical and socially-embedded response to our health and well-being needs.

One scholar who may, indirectly, provide a way of thinking about how – and why – to seed CBT within our communities and societies is Taleb (2012), whose focus of scholarship is what he terms "antifragility". Antifragility refers to the characteristics that allow systems to learn, grow and strengthen under conditions of hardship. In contrast to resilience, which is concerned with remaining strong (but fundamentally unchanged) in the face of difficulties, Taleb is interested in why certain systems actually thrive when confronted with unpredictable, high-impact events such as market crashes and pandemics.

Antifragility, according to Taleb, is a quality present in nature, including complex systems such as the human body. For example, placing a moderate amount of pressure on our muscles and joints through physical exercise results in small muscle tears. When the body repairs these small tears, we become stronger. The antifragility of the human body is also evident through the process of vaccination: by introducing controlled quantities of diseases into our bodies through immunisation our bodies build resistance to that disease. Thus, antifragile systems need disorder if they are to thrive. In relation to health and well-being, where this is denied us, we move into a state of decline. For example, our muscles will atrophy if they are not exposed to regular small tears of muscle fibre and a sedentary lifestyle actually increases the likelihood of long-term physical health conditions.

How the notion of antifragility applies to mental health and how CBT practitioners might facilitate this is yet to be explored. Nonetheless, it is implicit in the concept of post-traumatic growth (Joseph, 2012) and perhaps third wave approaches such as compassionate mind therapy (Gilbert, 2005).

Looking to the future, we anticipate an additional and repositioned role for CBT as a means in instilling antifragility in our community and social systems. This could be achieved through city-wide initiatives for meeting the mental health needs of the population. Increasingly, we are seeing initiatives beyond traditional mental health services to support communities.

This is a valuable trend and certainly expands the availability of support. For example, in 2007, The Center for Health and Health Care in Schools, in Washington, DC, recommended future directions in practices, policies and systems development based on a 16-month review of mental health programmes (Price & Lear, 2008). The review concluded that school-connected mental health was essential to effective schools and well-functioning mental health systems. A recognition of the role of schools in enabling mental health is increasingly influencing thinking in the UK (Department of Health and Social Care, 2017). There have also been city-wide initiatives in the USA (Price & Lear, 2008).

In the UK in 2017, the 'Thrive London' initiative was launched, drawing upon previous work conducted in New York. Thrive LDN is a city-wide movement whose goal is to improve the mental health and well-being of Londoners, and which engages in a range of activities and operations to change population outcomes. The initiative intentionally links mental health and a diverse range of social, economic and environmental factors that impact the populations. Thrive LDN is supported by the Mayor of London, the NHS, Public Health England, London borough councils and the Healthy London Partnership. Bringing together these diverse stakeholders highlights an awareness of how social disadvantage, risk exposure and social inequities play a fundamental role in poor health outcomes, and that these factors are influenced by the local and national distribution of power and resources which shape the conditions of daily life.

The recognition of how CBT knowledge might increase its sensitivity and acceptability to different social and cultural groups is also a topic of considerable current interest. The British Association for Behavioural & Cognitive Psychotherapies (BABCP), the Lead Organisation for CBT in the UK and Ireland, has produced a positive practice guide for creating more equitable access and outcomes for black, Asian and minority ethnic service users (Beck et al., 2019). It also delivers training and support for its members through the BABCP's Equality and Culture Special Interest Group. However, embedding CBT services within communities themselves is a wider issue.

Although beyond the scope of an introductory CBT text, it is important to recognise that the extent to which psychological interventions are sufficiently culturally sensitive to empower rather than marginalise is an ongoing debate. Ratele (2019), for example, has argued cogently that unless we are prepared to listen to and work directly with communities, we will not ultimately be able to understand the whole person who requests our help. Arguments such as these, and the initiatives that arise from them in bringing together faith communities, arts organisations, schools as well as health and social care, generate important questions for the CBT community. For example, in the spirit of Miller (1969), to what extent would the professional community wish to "give CBT away"? Clearly there is much that could be offered, for example, in training local volunteers to use trauma-informed work. Yet this would involve a fundamentally different and new direction for CBT, one that is centred on the notion of empowering communities rather than treating individuals.

Questions for theory, research and practice arising from this level include:

- What would antifragility look like in relation to our collective health and well-being? Which principles and methods emanating from CBT would be most relevant to building antifragility?
- How do we 'seed' CBT within our communities?
- How best can communities be trained to deliver CBT principles and methods and who would need to train them?
- What issues for credentialing and regulation arise from 'seeding' CBT in community settings?

Engaging effectively with wicked problems requires a willingness to embrace paradox and uncertainty (Rittel & Webber, 1973). The former can help us gain clarity about the origins of the issue of concern and the latter ensures that we remain open to emerging avenues of response that are potentially available (and the highly diverse sources from which these perspectives emerge).

In addition to considering how societies and the individuals within them may need to transform, grappling with wicked problems necessitates new approaches to exploring, conceptualising, researching and decision-making that draw upon a wider variety of investigative landscapes. The invitation from authors such as Brown et al. (2010) to explicitly draw upon our collective imaginative capability and the need to look across, rather than within, individual disciplines raises interesting possibilities for how we might respond to the mental health crisis and the role that CBT might play. This does not, of course, imply that we should reject the methods, tools and practices that have enabled CBT to make its existing, noteworthy contribution. Rather, we are proposing a need to remain radically open to new and diverse ideas, concepts and directions that reflect the reality of our times. This we see as being in keeping with the spirit of CBT itself – a field of which a hallmark feature is its willingness and ability to evolve in light of encountering new psychological puzzles, new data from our science and the demands of a new era.

Conclusion

CBT has come a long way from the early days when it was seen as applicable to a relatively limited range of clinical issues. The fact that the field has evolved does, we believe, attest to the fact that it is a thriving discipline. However, CBT is arguably yet to face its greatest challenge. Effectiveness in the decades ahead will need to look different from how we have defined effectiveness up until now and will take multiple forms as a function of the contexts in which CBT needs to be applied.

In reflecting on what could lie ahead, our speculations have led us to predict that the next stage in the evolution of CBT will involve developments at each of three levels: (1) those arising from the changing needs of the clients who seek our services, (2) those arising from the emerging needs of the workforce who deliver CBT interventions in an increasingly complex climate of service delivery, and (3) those arising from efforts to embed CBT within wider social and community systems. These three levels allow us to consider with fresh eyes where CBT has made the greatest difference to date, and to identify untapped areas of contribution that might create a better future. By engaging with the questions, challenges and possibilities that arise from each of these levels, we see an opportunity for a paradigm shift within CBT – one that builds on its successes in addressing the needs of our clients through assisting and nurturing antifragility in the transformation of our local, national and global communities. If CBT rises to this challenge, then, we believe, the future of the field is potentially limitless.

Reflective Activity: Enabling yourself for the world of tomorrow

In this chapter we have identified three levels that we believe represent important and promising directions for the future of CBT. Select the questions from one of these three levels. How would you answer these questions? How do you think that the CBT community, or the personal and professional communities with which you are engaged and perhaps more familiar, need to respond in order to meet the demands of a volatile, uncertain, complex and ambiguous world?

Interested in learning more? Check out …

Bannink, F. (2012). *Practicing positive CBT: From reducing distress to building success.* Chichester: Wiley-Blackwell.

Tehrani, N. (2011). *Managing trauma in the workplace: Supporting workers and organisations.* London: Routledge.

Taleb, N. N. (2012). *Antifragile: Things that gain from disorder.* London: Penguin.

Note

1 Rates of prevalence and incidence vary as a function of how mental health problems are defined, the methods used to measure the presence of disorder and cultural differences in the self-reporting of distress. They also vary as a function of how recently the data were collected. These statistics are best understood, therefore, as illustrative rather than providing definitive statements on specific numbers of individuals directly living with a mental health problem at any given point in time.

Conclusion

Throughout this book, we have explored CBT as a well-regarded and efficacious intervention for a range of emotional and psychological difficulties for both adults and children. In recent years, it has increasingly been seen as the treatment of choice for a variety of mental health diagnoses. Beyond mental health we have provided some other examples of interventions for non-diagnosable psychological dilemmas and problems of living. As is evident through the burgeoning number of self-help books and online tools, CBT-based solutions are now offered for a diversity of human concerns and we would see this trend as likely to continue in the years ahead.

In the spirit of experiential learning which lies at the heart of CBT, we started the book by asking you to consider the principles and methods that you would be reading about and how you might apply them to aspects of your own life and work. Throughout the book we have sought to illustrate how CBT aims to equip people with a way of understanding their needs and a technology that they can use to support themselves. Becoming effective in the use of CBT means that all those who deliver it also have a process they can use to navigate periods of challenge, change and opportunity in their own lives. Suggesting that you approach reading the book with a purpose in mind has been a way of personalising your journey and, where appropriate, experimenting with the ideas.

By way of drawing the book to a close, we invite you to revisit your original thoughts about what you hoped to gain from reading this book and to what extent your objectives have been realised. To assist in this endeavour, we have provided you with a reflective tool. The value of using reflective tools to guide learning and development has been described elsewhere (e.g. Lane & Corrie, 2006; Corrie et al., 2016). They take the form of a series of questions that help you to draw together your thoughts and consider plans for future learning. For the purposes of this book, we recommend that you use the questions provided creatively and repeatedly, that you share your ideas with partners, colleagues and peers, and, if you are currently studying, with your supervisors and trainers.

Reflective Activity: Your reflective tool

1. What have been the main things that you have learned about CBT through reading this book? You may find it helpful to use the following prompts:
    o   What was already familiar to you?
    o   What was new to you?
    o   What, if anything, surprised you?
    o   Did you hold any myths about CBT that this book has challenged? If so, what were they and what do you believe now that is different?
2. Which ideas presented in the book have been most impactful for you personally and professionally?
    o   Of those ideas that have had the greatest impact, can you identify what made them so persuasive?
    o   Can you identify any ways in which these ideas might be applied to a specific area of your life or professional practice?
    o   Can you identify any way in which the principles and methods could be relevant to a challenge you have faced?
3. What have you learned about your own cognitive world: that is, your automatic thoughts, assumptions, standards, beliefs and images?
    o   What is working well?
    o   What might benefit from some changes?
    o   How might you make those changes?
    o   Are there any reasoning biases which you have acknowledged that could be challenged?
    o   Can you make any connections between how you feel and think in different situations?
4. What have you learned about your own behaviour?
    o   What is working well?
    o   What might benefit from some changes?
    o   Are there behaviours you wish to increase, decrease or instil?
    o   How might you make some of those changes?
    o   Can you make any connections between how you feel and act in different situations?
5. If you needed help from a therapist, would you select CBT as your therapy of choice?
    o   If so, why? If not, why not?
    o   If your response is dependent, what are the relevant factors?

○   What does this book suggest to you about who is most and least suited to CBT and why?

○   Would you recommend CBT to a friend who needed psychological support?

6.   What areas have piqued your interest enough to want to learn more?

○   Which of the suggestions for future reading have intrigued you?

○   What further reading will you attempt?

○   There are lots of introductory courses available – which might you explore?

○   Would you be interested in further training? If so, what qualifications might you wish to pursue?

A final word

CBT is a growing family of approaches to mental health and well-being. It strives to build on an evidence base and is a collaborative enterprise between clients and practitioners. It also increasingly enables self-help and healthier living.

We hope that we have conveyed some of the excitement we feel about this work, but also that we have indicated the need to always adopt a reflective and enquiring approach to ideas. As practitioners, we have worked in the field for several decades and have seen many changes which have led to a refinement of the offer that CBT is able to make to health, well-being and social change. We have seen CBT emerge from a marginal and often contested activity to become a robustly mainstream approach.

However, although the widespread appeal of CBT is clear, popularity is not synonymous with understanding and knowledge. What matters is accessibility. In his Reith lecture, acclaimed musician Daniel Barenboim (2006: 82) stated that, "Accessibility does not come through populism, accessibility comes through more interest and more knowledge". If this book has helped you to acquire a little more of each, and inspired you to read further, then we have achieved our purpose.

We continue our journey into learning more about this fascinating specialism and wish you well as you continue yours.

Sarah and David

References

Bandura, A. (1971). *Social learning theory*. New York: General Learning Press.

Bannink, F. (2012). *Practicing positive CBT: From reducing distress to building success*. Chichester: Wiley-Blackwell.

Barber, H. F. (1992). Developing strategic leadership: the US army war college experience. *Journal of Management Development, 11*, 4–12.

Barenboim, D. (2006). In the beginning was sound. Reproduced in *Remarkable Minds: A celebration of the Reith Lectures BBC Radio 4*. London: Headline Publishing Group.

Baucom, D. H., Fischer, M. S., Worrell, M., Corrie, S., Belus, J. M., Molyva, E., & Boeding, S. E. (2018). Couple-based intervention for depression: An effectiveness study in the National Health Service in England. *Family Process, 57*(2), 275–292. doi: 10.1111/famp.12332.

Baucom, D. H., Fischer, M. S., Corrie, S., Worrell, M., & Boeding, S. E. (2020). *Treating relationship distress and psychopathology in couples: A cognitive-behavioural approach*. Abingdon, UK: Routledge.

Beck, A., Naz, S., Brooks, M., & Jankowska, M. (2019). *Improving access to psychological therapies (IAPT): Black, Asian and minority ethnic service user positive practice guided 2019*. Bury, UK: British Association for Behavioural & Cognitive Psychotherapies.

Beck, A. T., Rush, A. J., Shaw, B. F., & Emery, G. (1979). *Cognitive therapy of depression*. New York: Guilford Press.

Beck, J. S. (2011). *Cognitive behavior therapy: Basics and beyond* (2nd ed.). New York: Guilford Press.

Beck, J. S. (2020). *Cognitive behavior therapy: Basics and beyond* (3rd ed.). New York: Guilford Press.

Bennett-Levy, J. (2019). Why therapists should walk the talk: the theoretical and empirical case for personal practice in therapist training and professional development. *Journal of Behavior Therapy and Experimental Psychiatry, 62*, 133–145.

Bennett-Levy, J., Butler, G., Fennell, M., Hackmann, A., Mueller, M., & Westbrook, D. (2004). *Oxford guide to behavioural experiments in cognitive therapy*. Oxford: Oxford University Press.

Boulton, J. G., Allen, P. M., & Bowman, C. (2015). *Embracing complexity: Strategic perspectives for an age of turbulence*. Oxford: Oxford University Press.

Bradbury, K. (2016). Mohammad: a case study of depression using behavioural activation. In S. Corrie, M. J. Townend, & A. Cockx (Eds.), *Assessment and case formulation in cognitive behavioural therapy* (2nd ed.). London: SAGE.

Brown, V. A., Harris, J. A., & Russell, J. Y. (2010). *Tackling wicked problems through the transdisciplinary imagination*. London: Earthscan.

Bruch, M. (2015). *Beyond diagnosis: Case formulation in cognitive behavioural therapy* (2nd ed.). Chichester: Wiley Blackwell.

Butler, G., Fennell, M., & Hackmann, A. (2008). *Cognitive behavioural therapy for anxiety disorders: Mastering clinical challenges*. New York: Guilford Press.

Cavanagh, M. J., & Lane, D. (2012). Coaching psychology coming of age: the challenges we face in the messy world of complexity. *International Coaching Psychology Review*, 7, 75–90.

Clark, D. M., & Wells, A. (1995). A cognitive model of social phobia. In R. G. Heimberg, M. R. Liebowitz, D. A. Hope, & F. R. Schneider (Eds.), *Social phobia: Diagnosis, assessment and treatment*. New York: Guilford Press.

Corrie, S., & Lane, D. A. (2010). *Constructing stories, telling tales: A guide to formulation in applied psychology*. London: Karnac.

Corrie, S., & Parsons, A. (in press). Emerging conversations about the role of coaching in mental health. In M. Watts & I. Florance (Eds.), *Emerging conversations in coaching*. Hove, UK: Routledge.

Corrie, S., Townend, M. J., & Cockx, A. (2016). *Assessment and case formulation in cognitive behavioural therapy* (2nd ed.). London: SAGE.

David, D., Cristea, I., & Hofmann, S. G. (2018). Why cognitive behavioral therapy is the current gold standard of psychotherapy. *Frontiers in Psychiatry*, 9(4), 1–3.

de Bono, E. (2006). The scientist practitioner as thinker: a comment on judgment and design. In D. A. Lane & S. Corrie (Eds.), *The modern scientist practitioner: A guide to practice in psychology*. Hove, UK: Routledge.

Demsky, K., & Mack, L. (2008). Environmental design research (EDR): the field of study and guide to the literature. *Journal of Architectural and Planning Research*, 25(4), 271–275.

Department of Health (2008). *Improving access to psychological therapies – implementation plan: National guidelines for regional delivery*. London: Department of Health.

Department of Health and Social Care (DHSC) & Department for Education (DfE) (2017). *Transforming children and young people's mental health provision: A green paper*. London: Department of Health and Social Care.

Doom, J. R., & Gunnar, M. R. (2015). Stress in infancy and early childhood: effects on development. In J. D. Wright (Ed.), *International encyclopedia of the social & behavioral sciences* (2nd ed.). Oxford: Elsevier.

Eysenck, H. J., & Martin, I. (1987). *Theoretical foundations of behaviour therapy*. New York: Pergamon.

Fenn, K., & Byrne, M. (2008). The key principles of cognitive behavioural therapy. *InnovAiT*, 6(9), 579–585. Retrieved from: https://journals.sagepub.com/doi/pdf/10.1177/1755738012471029.

Foa, E. B., Yadin, E., & Lichner, T. K. (2012). *Exposure and response (ritual) prevention for obsessive-compulsive disorder: Therapist guide* (2nd ed.). Oxford: Oxford University Press.

Gaudiano, B. (2008). Cognitive-behavioral therapies: achievements and challenges. *Evidence-Based Mental Health*, 11(1), 5–7.

Gendlin, E. T. (1996). *Focusing-oriented psychotherapy: A manual of the experiential method*. New York: Guilford Press.

Gilbert, P. (2005). *Compassion: Conceptualisations, research and use in psychotherapy*. Hove, UK: Routledge.

Goldiamond, I. (2002). Toward a constructional approach to social problems: ethical and constitutional issues raised by applied behavior analysis. *Behavior and Social Issues*, 11(2), 108–197.

Green, H., Mcginnity, A., Ford, T., & Goodman, R. (2005). *Mental health of children and young people in Great Britain 2004*. Basingstoke, UK: Palgrave Macmillan.

Greenberger, D., & Padesky, C. A. (2015). *Mind over mood* (2nd ed.). New York: Guilford Press.

Hayes, S. C. (2004). Acceptance and commitment therapy, relational frame theory and the third wave of behavioral and cognitive therapies. *Behaviour Therapy*, *35*, 639–665.

Hofmann, S. G., & Asmundson, G. J. G. (2008). Acceptance and mindfulness-based therapy: new wave or old hat? *Clinical Psychology Review*, *28*(1), 1–16.

Hofmann, S. G., Asnaani, A., Vonk, I. J. J., Swayer, A. T., & Fang, A. (2012). The efficacy of cognitive behavioral therapy: a review of meta-analyses. *Cognitive Therapy Research*, *36*(5), 427–440.

Jones, M. C. (1924). A laboratory study of fear: the case of Peter. *Pedagogical Seminary*, *31*, 308–315. Retrieved from: http://psychclassics.yorku.ca/Jones/

Jones, M. C. (1926). The development of early behavior patterns in young children. *Pedagogical Seminary*, *33*, 537–585.

Joseph, S. (2012). *What doesn't kill us: The new psychology of posttraumatic growth*. New York: Basic Books.

Kazdin, A. (2012). *The token economy: A review and evaluation*. New York: Springer.

Kelly, G.A. (1955). *The psychology of personal constructs: A theory of personality*. London: Routledge.

Kennerley, H., Kirk, J., & Westbrook, D. (2017). *An introduction to cognitive behaviour therapy: Skills and applications* (3rd ed.). London: SAGE.

King's Fund, (The) (2020). *Long term medical conditions and multi-morbidity*. Retrieved from: www.kingsfund.org.uk/projects/time-think-differently/trends-disease-and-disability-long-term-conditions-multi-morbidity.

Kovacs, L., & Corrie, S. (2017). Executive coaching in an era of complexity. Study 1: Does executive coaching work and if so why? A Realist Evaluation. *International Coaching Psychology Review*, *12*(2), 194–209.

Krasner, L. (1980). *Environmental design and human behavior: A psychology of the individual in society*. New York: Pergamon.

Kuyken, W., Padesky, C. A., & Dudley, R. (2009). *Collaborative case conceptualization: Working effectively with clients in cognitive-behavioral therapy*. New York: Guilford Press.

Lane, D. A. (1975). *The guidance centre: A new approach to childhood difficulties*. London: The King's Fund.

Lane, D. A. (1978). *The impossible child* (Vols 1 & 2). London: ILEA.

Lane, D. A. (1990). *The impossible child*. Stoke-on-Trent, UK: Trentham Books.

Lane, D. A., & Corrie, S. (2006). *The modern scientist-practitioner: A guide to practice in psychology*. Hove, UK: Routledge.

Lane, D. A., & Corrie, S. (2015). Case formulation as a process of building a story that makes sense for the therapist and the client. In M. Bruch (Ed.), *Beyond diagnosis: Case formulation in cognitive behavioural therapy* (2nd ed.). Chichester, UK: Wiley.

Lee, D. (2005). The perfect nurturer: a model to develop a compassionate mind within the context of cognitive therapy. In P. Gilbert (Ed.), *Compassion: Conceptualisations, research and use in psychotherapy*. Hove, UK: Brunner-Routledge.

Martell, C. R., Dimidjian, S., & Herman-Dunn, R. (2013). *Behavioural activation for depression: A clinician's guide*. New York: Guilford Press.

McKay M., Davis, M., & Fanning, P. (2011). *Thoughts & feelings: Taking control of your moods & your life* (4th ed.). Oakland, CA: New Harbinger Publications.

McKay, M., Wood, J. C., & Brantley, J. (2007). *The dialectical behavior therapy skills workbook*. Oakland, CA: New Harbinger Publications.

McManus, S., Bebbington, P., Jenkins, R., & Brugha, T. (2016). *Mental health and wellbeing in England: Adult psychiatric morbidity survey 2004*. Leeds: NHS Digital.

McNamee, S., & Gergen, K. J. (1992). *Therapy as social construction*. London: SAGE.

Mead, G. H. (1932). *The philosophy of the present*. LaSalle, IL: Open Court.

Meichenbaum, D. (1976). *Cognitive behavior modification*. New York: Plenum Press.

Meyer, V. (1966). Modification of expectations in cases with obsessive rituals. *Behaviour Research and Therapy, 4*(4), 273–280.

Miller, G. A. (1969). Psychology as a means of promoting human welfare. *American Psychologist, 24*, 1063–1075.

Morrison, A. P., Renton, J. C., Dunn, H., Williams, S., & Bentall, R. P. (2003). *Cognitive therapy for psychosis: A formulation-based approach*. Hove, UK: Brunner-Routledge.

National Collaborating Centre for Mental Health (2019). *The improving access to psychological therapies manual*. Retrieved from: www.england.nhs.uk/publication/the-improving-access-to-psychological-therapies-manual/.

NHS England (2014, October). *NHS Five Year Forward Review*. London: NHS England. Retrieved from: www.england.nhs.uk/publication/nhs-five-year-forward-view/.

NICE (2004a). *Anxiety: Management of anxiety (panic disorder, with and without agoraphobia, and generalised anxiety disorder) in adults in primary, secondary and community care*. Clinical guideline CG22. London: National Institute for Health and Clinical Excellence. Retrieved from: www.nice.org.uk/guidance/CG22.

NICE (2004b). *Depression: Management of depression in primary and secondary care*. Clinical guideline CG23. London: National Institute for Health and Clinical Excellence. Retrieved from: www.nice.org.uk/guidance/CG23.

NICE (2005). *Obsessive compulsive disorder: Core interventions in the treatment of obsessive compulsive disorder and body dysmorphic disorder*. Clinical guideline CG31. Retrieved from: www.nice.org.uk/guidance/CG31.

NICE (2009). *Depression in adults: Recognition and management*. Clinical guideline CG90. Retrieved from: www.nice.org.uk/guidance/CG90.

NICE (2011). *Common mental health disorders: Identification and pathways to care*. Clinical Guideline CG123. London: National Institute for Health and Clinical Excellence. Retrieved from: www.nice.org.uk/guidance/CG123.

NICE (2019). *Evidence-based research on cognitive behaviour therapy*. Retrieved from: www.evidence. nhs.uk/search?q=NICE+cognitive+behavioural +therapy.

O'Leary, K. D., & O'Leary, S. G. (1972). *Classroom management: The successful use of behavior modification*. New York: Pergamon.

Padesky, C. (1993). *Socratic questioning: Changing minds or guiding discovery?* Keynote address delivered at the European Association for Behavioural & Cognitive Therapies Conference, London, September.

Padesky, C. (1994). Schema change processes in cognitive therapy. *Clinical Psychology and Psychotherapy, 1*, 267–278.

Padesky, C. (2005). *Constructing a new self: Cognitive therapy for personality disorders*. Workshop presented in London, 23–24 May.

Pereira, J., Barkham, M., Kellett, S., & Saxon, D. (2017). The role of practitioner resilience and mindfulness in effective practice: a practice-based feasibility study. *Administration and Policy in Mental Health and Mental Health Services Research, 44*, 691–704.

Persons, J. B. (2012). *The case formulation approach to cognitive behavior therapy*. New York: Guilford Press.

Persons, J. B., & Davidson, J. (2010). Cognitive-behavioral case formulation. In K. S. Dobson (Ed.), *Handbook of cognitive behavioral therapies* (3rd ed.). New York: Guilford Press.

Premack, D. (1959). Toward empirical behavior laws: I. Positive reinforcement. *Psychological Review*, 66(4), 219–233.

Price, O. A., & Lear, J. G. (2008). *School mental health services for the 21st century: lessons from the District of Columbia School Mental Health Program.* Retrieved from: www.eric.ed.gov.

Ratele, K. (2019). *The world looks like this from here: Thoughts on African psychology.* Johannesburg, South Africa: Wits University Press.

Rittel, H., & Webber, M. (1973). Dilemmas in a general theory of planning. *Policy Sciences, 4,* 155–169.

Roth, A., & Fonagy, P. (2005). *What works for whom? A critical review of psychotherapy research* (2nd ed.). New York: Guilford Press.

Rutter, M., Tizard, J., Yule, W., Graham, P., & Whitmore, K. (1976). Isle of Wight studies, 1964–1974. *Psychological Medicine, 6*(2), 313–332.

Spence, S. H. (2003). Social skills training with children and young people: theory, evidence and practice. *Child and Adolescent Mental Health, 8*(2), 84–96.

Spiegler, M. D. (2015). *Contemporary behaviour therapy* (6th ed.). Boston, MA: Cengage Learning.

Stacey, R. D. (2010). *Complexity and organizational reality: Uncertainty and the need to rethink management after the collapse of investment capitalism* (2nd ed.). Abingdon, UK: Routledge.

Staddon, J. E. R., & Cerutti, D. T. (2003). Operant conditioning. *Annual Review of Psychology, 54,* 115–144.

Taleb, N. N. (2012). *Antifragile: Things that gain from disorder.* London: Penguin

Tehrani, N. (2011). *Managing trauma in the workplace: Supporting workers and organisations.* London: Routledge.

Tehrani, N., & Lane, D. A. (in press). The role for coaching in psychological trauma: emerging conversations about the role of coaching in mental health. In M. Watts & I. Florance (Eds.), *Emerging conversations in coaching.* Hove, UK: Routledge.

Thrive LDN. *Website.* Retrieved from: https://thriveldn.co.uk/.

Trower, P., & Hollin, C. R. (2016). *Handbook of social skills training: Clinical applications and new directions* (Vol. 2). Oxford: Pergamon Press.

Vos, T., Barber, R. M., Bell, B., Bertozzi-Villa, A., Biryukov, S., Bolliger, I., ... Dicker, D. (2015). Global, regional, and national incidence, prevalence, and years lived with disability for 301 acute and chronic diseases and injuries in 188 countries, 1990–2013: a systematic analysis for the global burden of disease study 2013. *The Lancet, 386*(9995), 743–800.

Welsh Assembly Government (2012). *Practical approaches to behaviour management in the classroom: A handbook for classroom teachers in primary schools.* Cardiff: Welsh Assembly Government.

Wolever, R. Q., Simmons, L. A., Sforzo, G. A., Dill, D., Kaye, M., Bechard, E. M., ... Yang, N. (2013). A systematic review of the literature on health and wellness coaching: defining a key behavioral intervention in healthcare. *Global Advances in Health and Medicine, 2*(4) 38–57.

World Health Organisation (2001). *World health report: Mental disorders affect one in four people.* Geneva: WHO. Retrieved from: www.who.int/whr/2001/media_centre/press-release/en/.

World Health Organisation (2003). *Caring for children and adolescents with mental disorders: Setting WHO directions*. Geneva: WHO. Retrieved from: www.who.int/mental_health/media/en/785.pdf.

World Health Organisation (2019). *Mental health of older adults*. Geneva: WHO. Retrieved from: www.who.int/en/news-room/ fact-sheets/detail/mental-health-of-older-adults.

Zube, E. H., & Moore, G. T. (1991). *Advances in environment, behaviour and design*. New York: Plenum.

Index